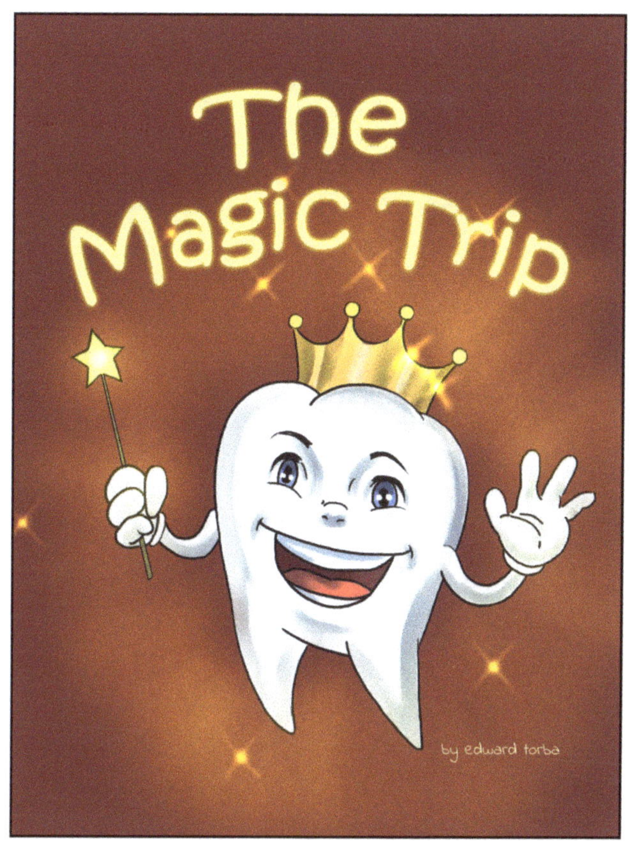

The Magic Trip

Copyright 2020 by Edward Torba

3rd Edition, revised

Originally released in 1977 as King Molar. Revised in 1988 and released as The Magic Trip

Published by: All Points Press

ISBN 978-1-7339161-1-0 (Hardcover)
ISBN 978-0-9850827-9-6 (Paperback)
ISBN 978-1-7339161-0-3 (e-Book)

Printed in the United States

Cover Design by S.C. Watson, www.oreganoproductions.com
Interior Design by The Deliberate Page, www.DeliberatePage.com
Illustrations by Arif Saputra

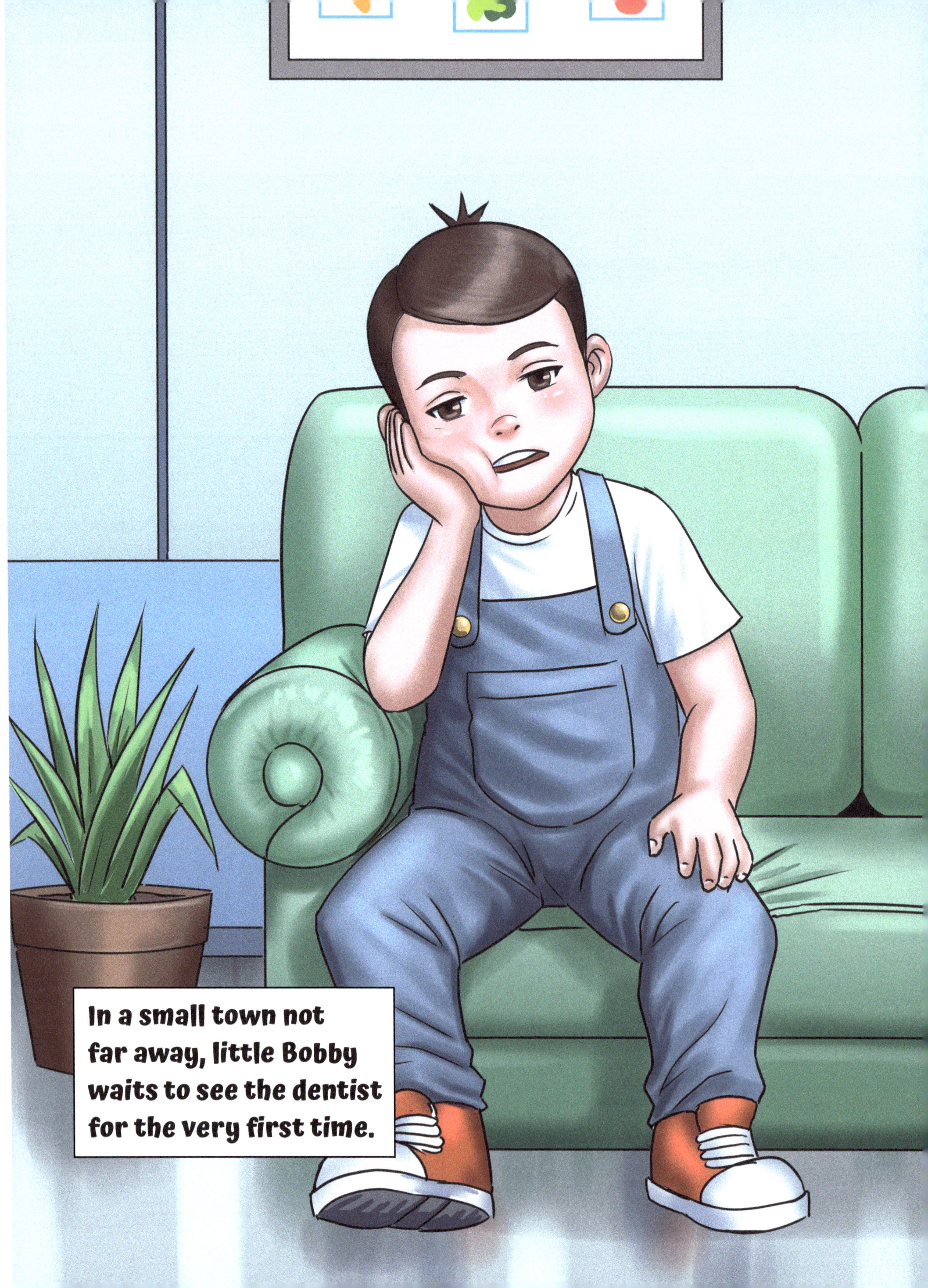

In a small town not far away, little Bobby waits to see the dentist for the very first time.

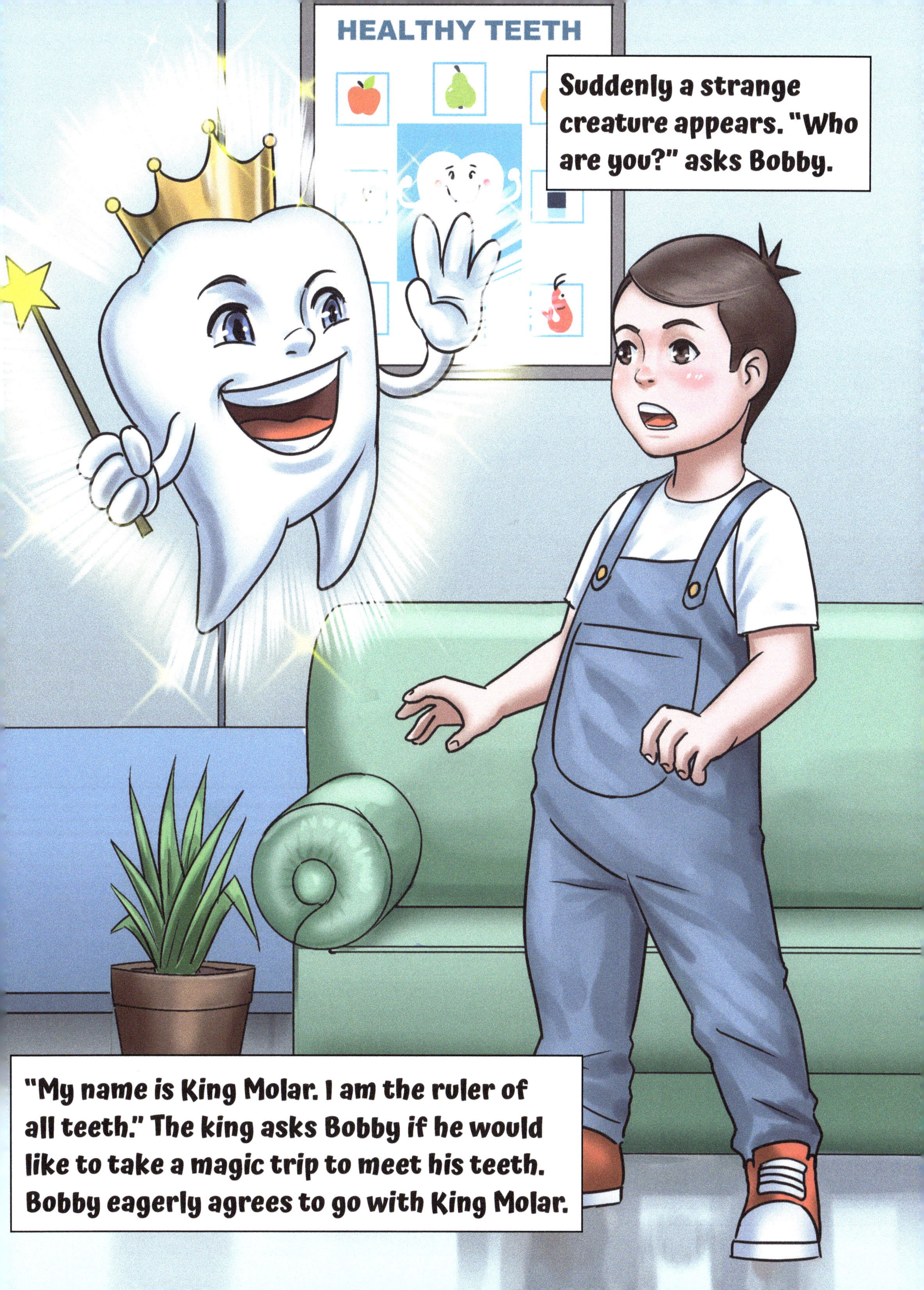

HEALTHY TEETH
Suddenly a strange creature appears. "Who are you?" asks Bobby.
"My name is King Molar. I am the ruler of all teeth." The king asks Bobby if he would like to take a magic trip to meet his teeth. Bobby eagerly agrees to go with King Molar.

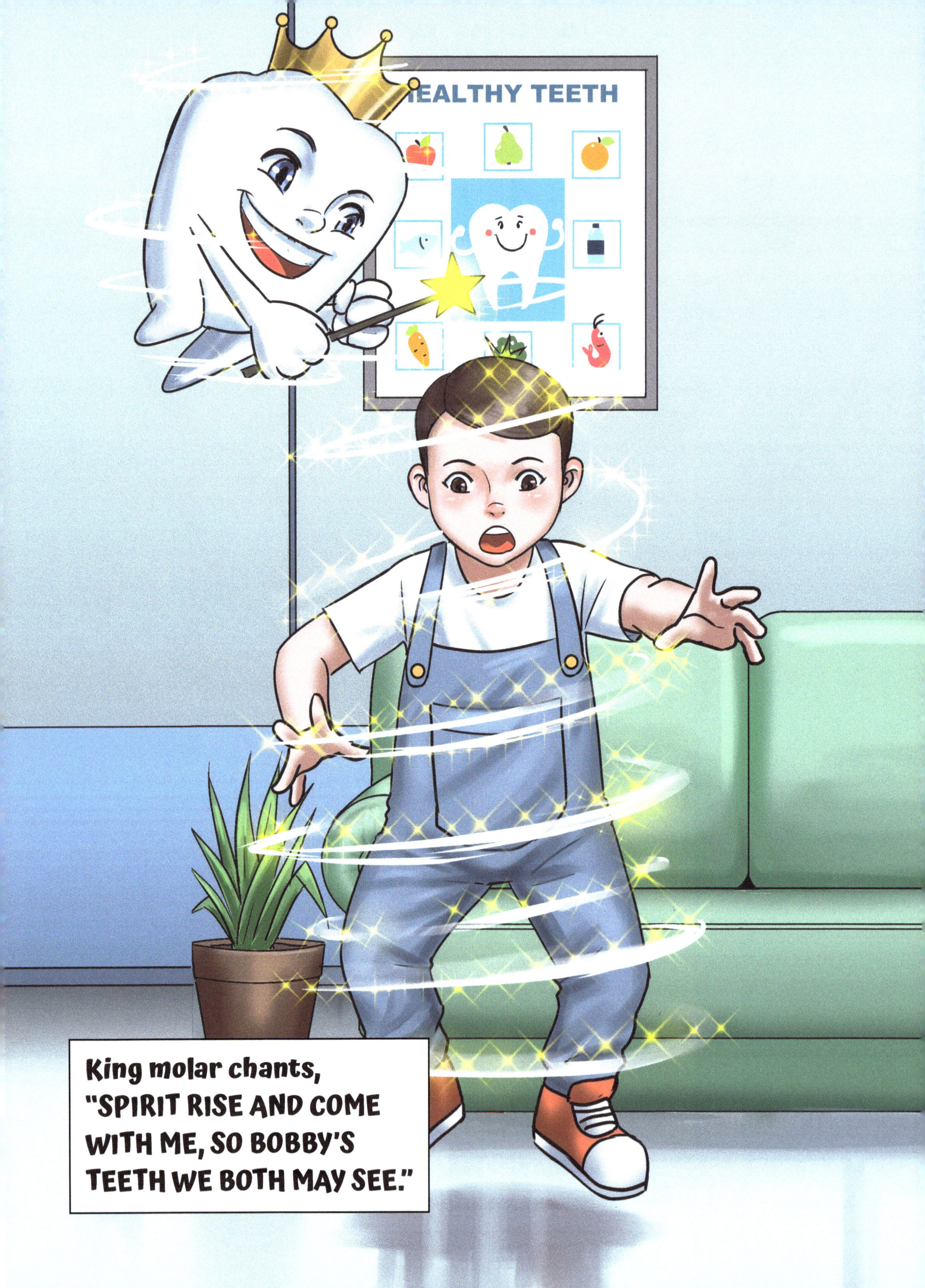
HEALTHY TEETH
King molar chants,
"SPIRIT RISE AND COME
WITH ME, SO BOBBY'S
TEETH WE BOTH MAY SEE."

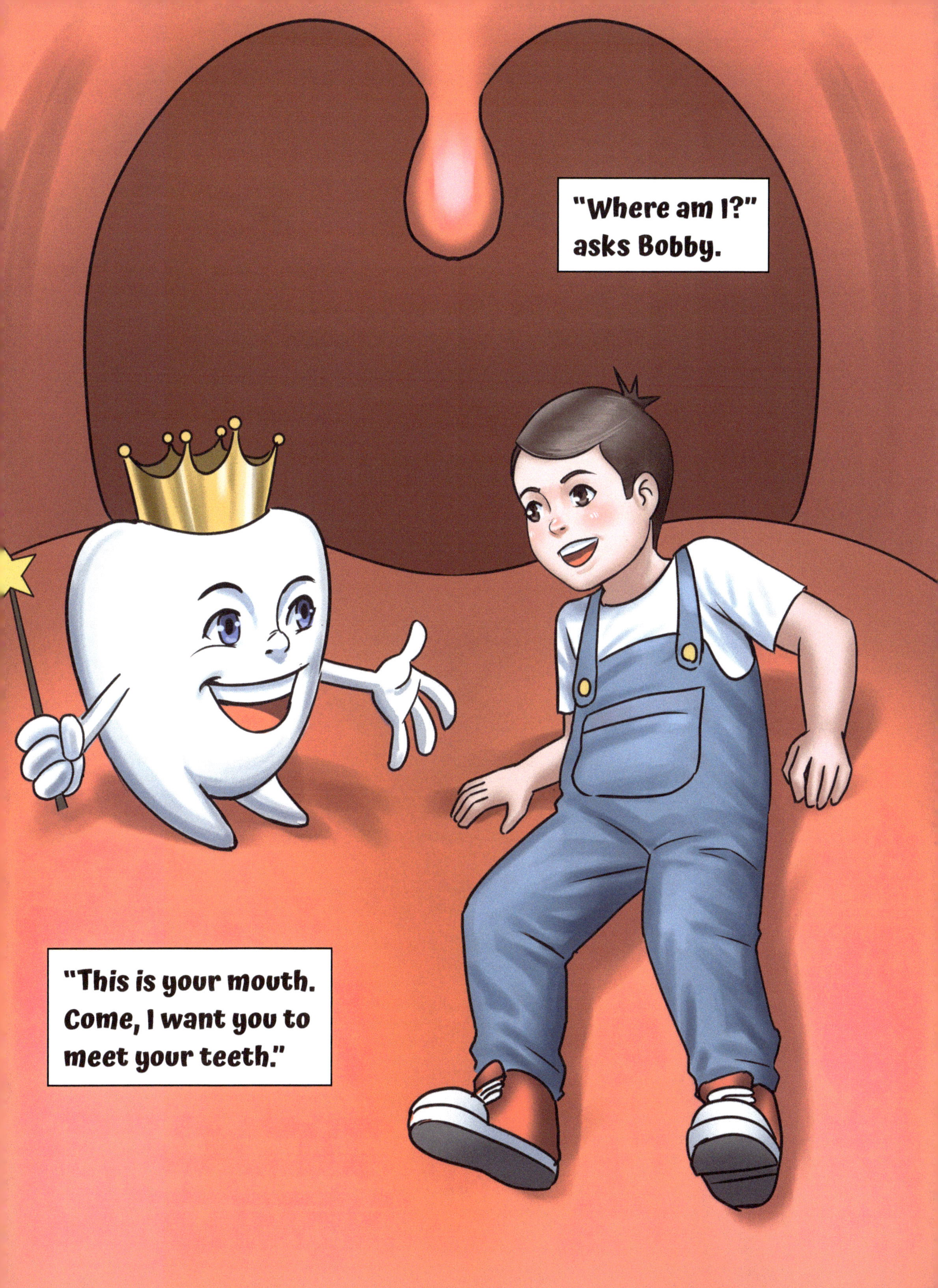

"Where am I?" asks Bobby.
"This is your mouth. Come, I want you to meet your teeth."

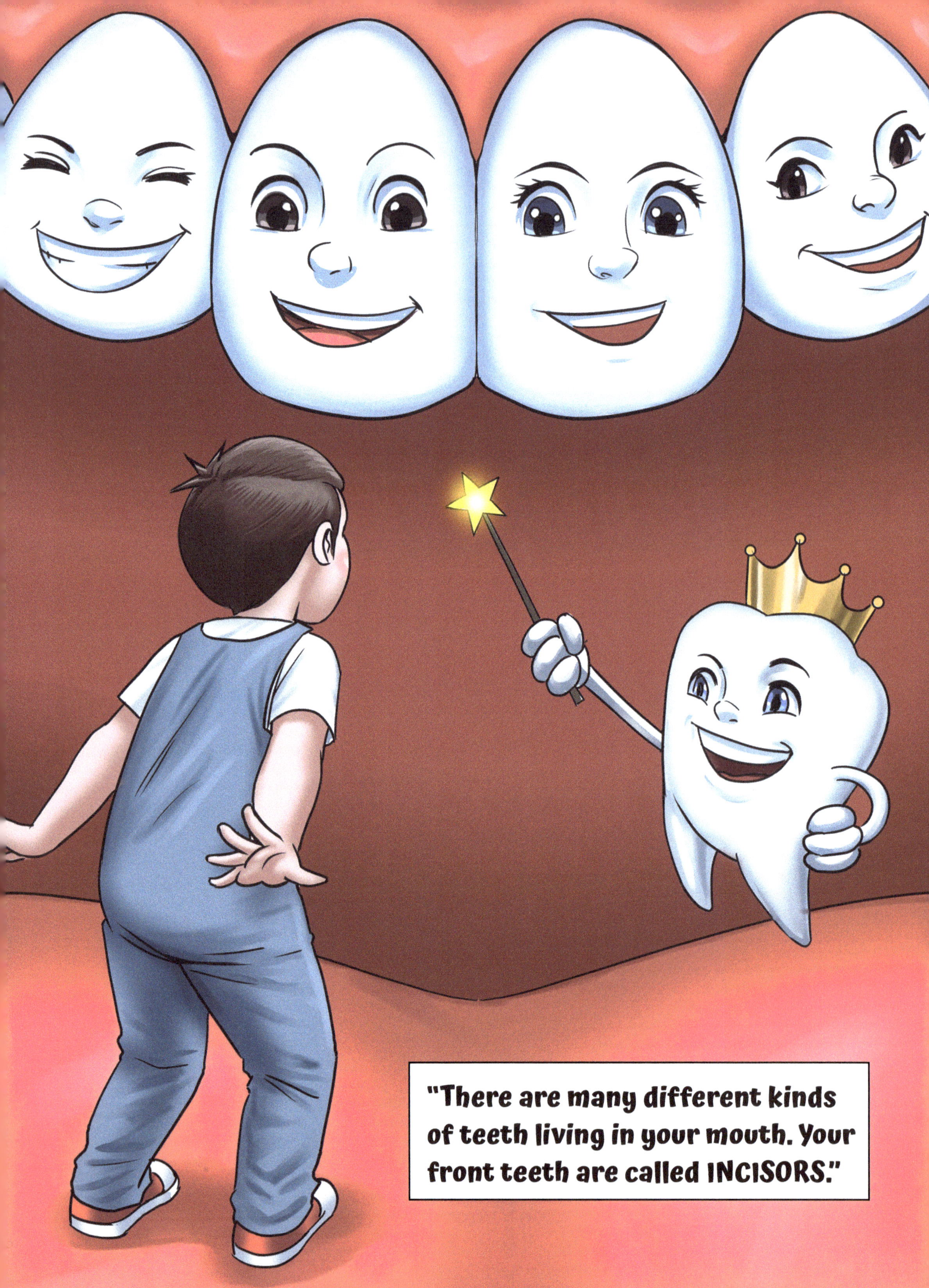
"There are many different kinds of teeth living in your mouth. Your front teeth are called INCISORS."

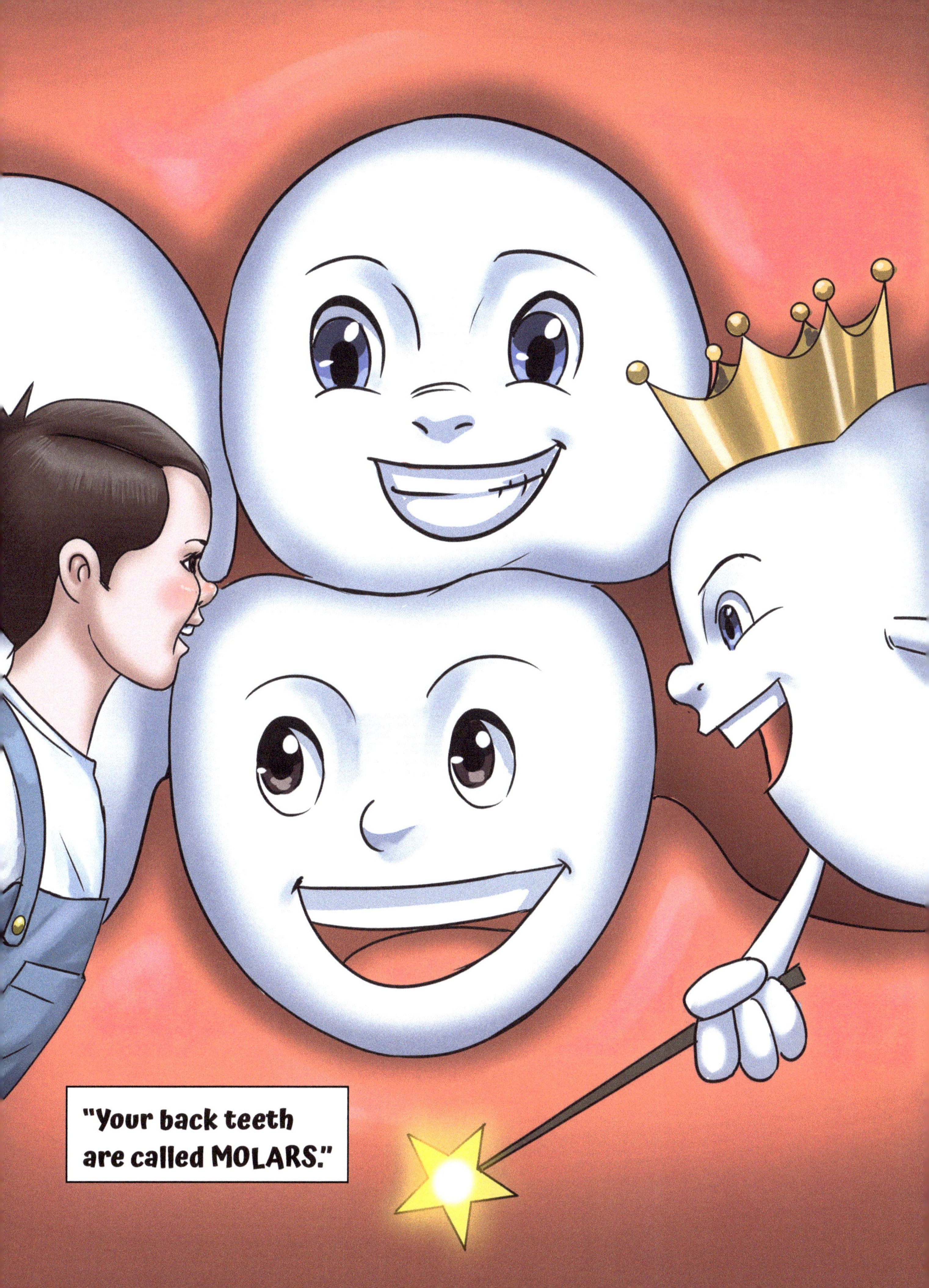

"Your back teeth
are called MOLARS."

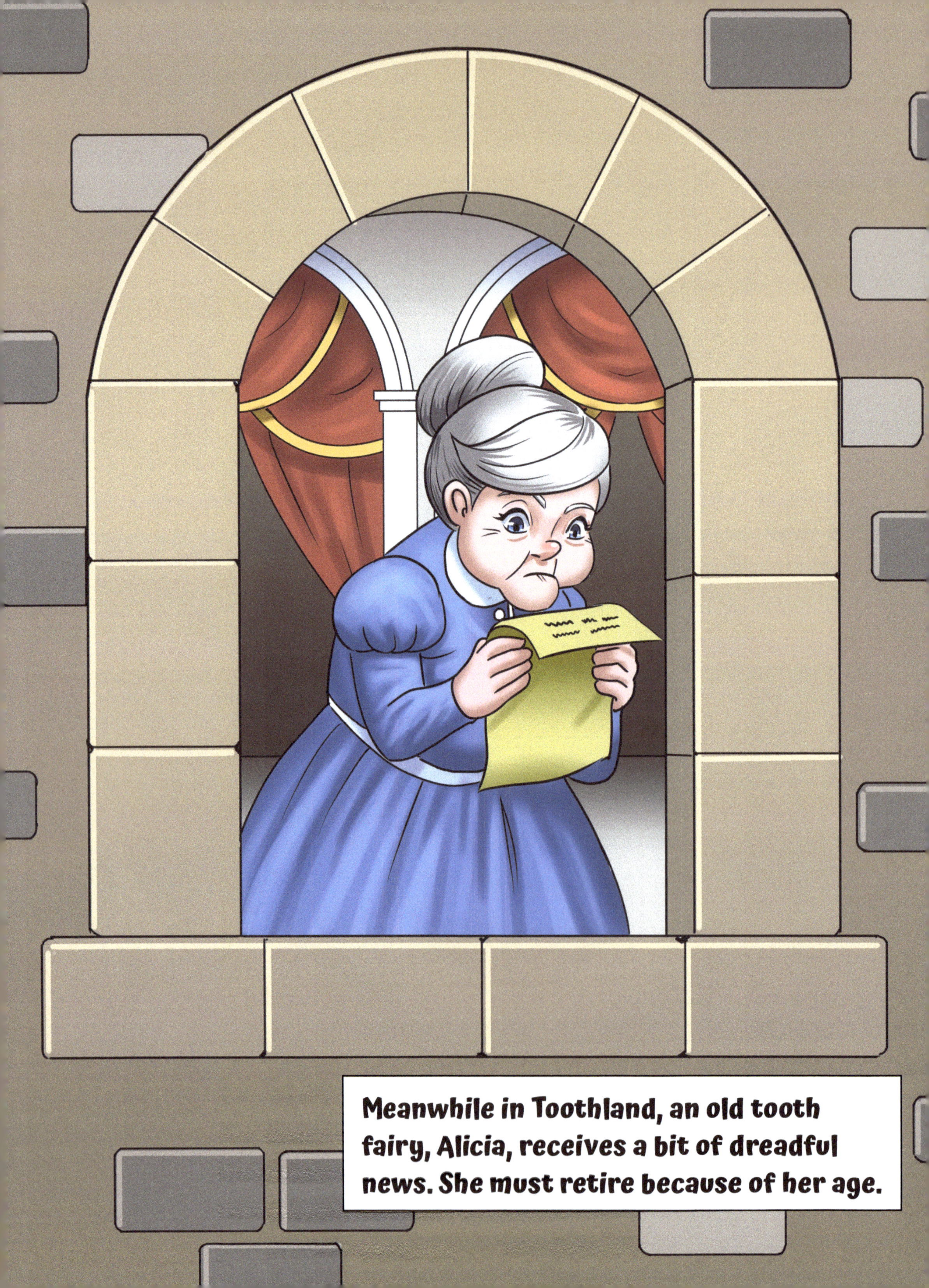

Meanwhile in Toothland, an old tooth fairy, Alicia, receives a bit of dreadful news. She must retire because of her age.

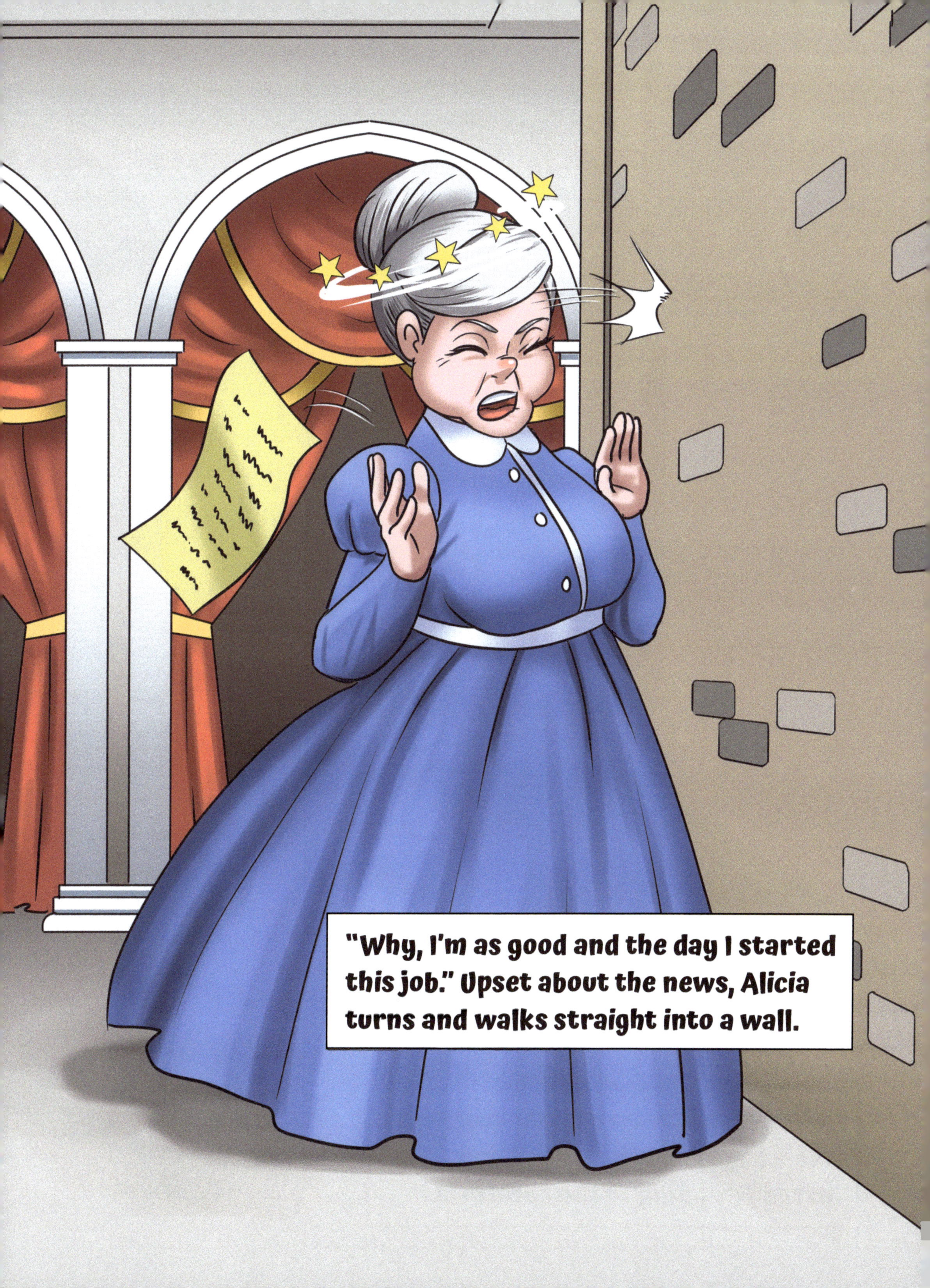

"Why, I'm as good and the day I started this job." Upset about the news, Alicia turns and walks straight into a wall.

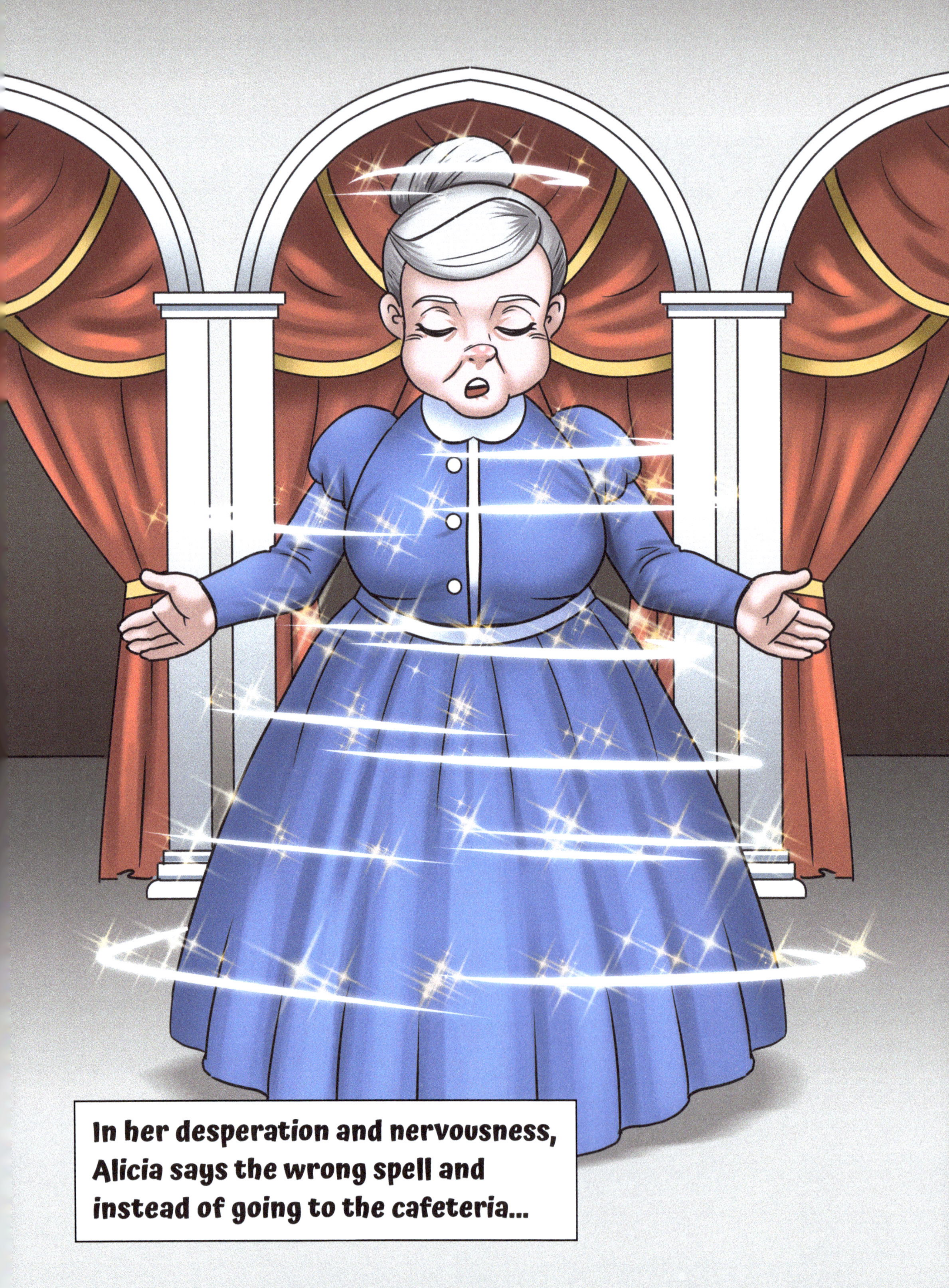

In her desperation and nervousness,
Alicia says the wrong spell and
instead of going to the cafeteria...

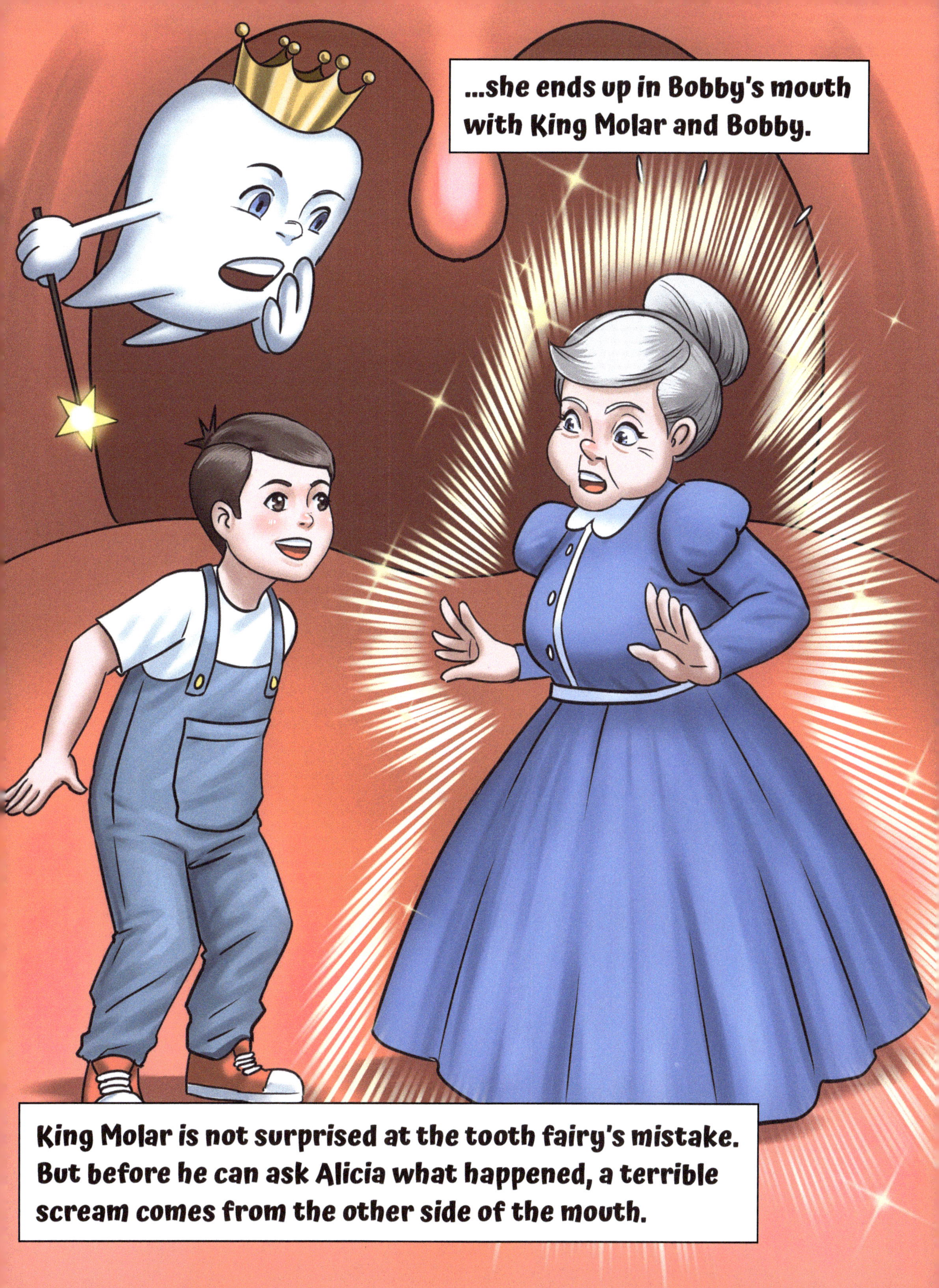

King Molar is not surprised at the tooth fairy's mistake. But before he can ask Alicia what happened, a terrible scream comes from the other side of the mouth.

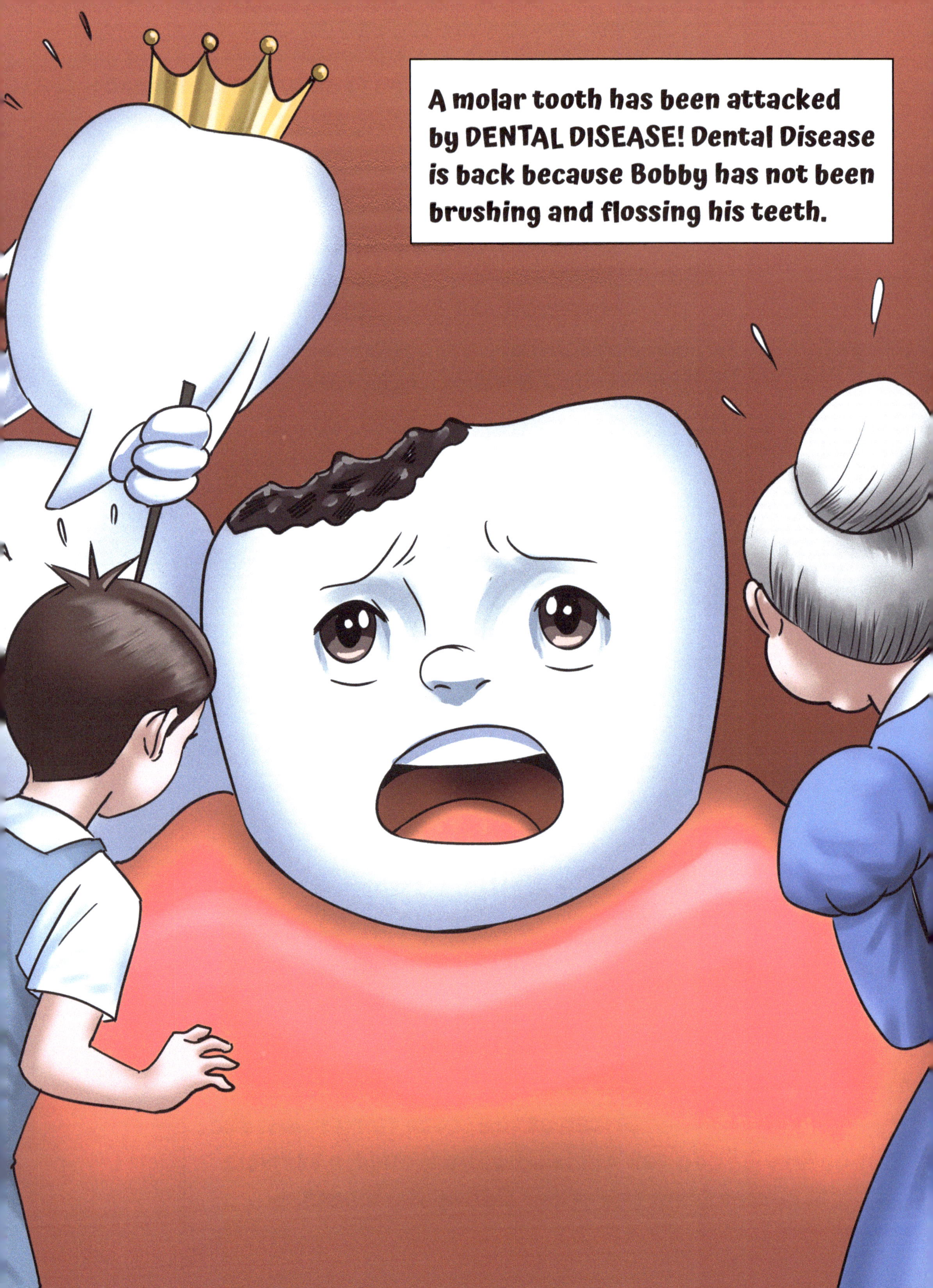
A molar tooth has been attacked by DENTAL DISEASE! Dental Disease is back because Bobby has not been brushing and flossing his teeth.

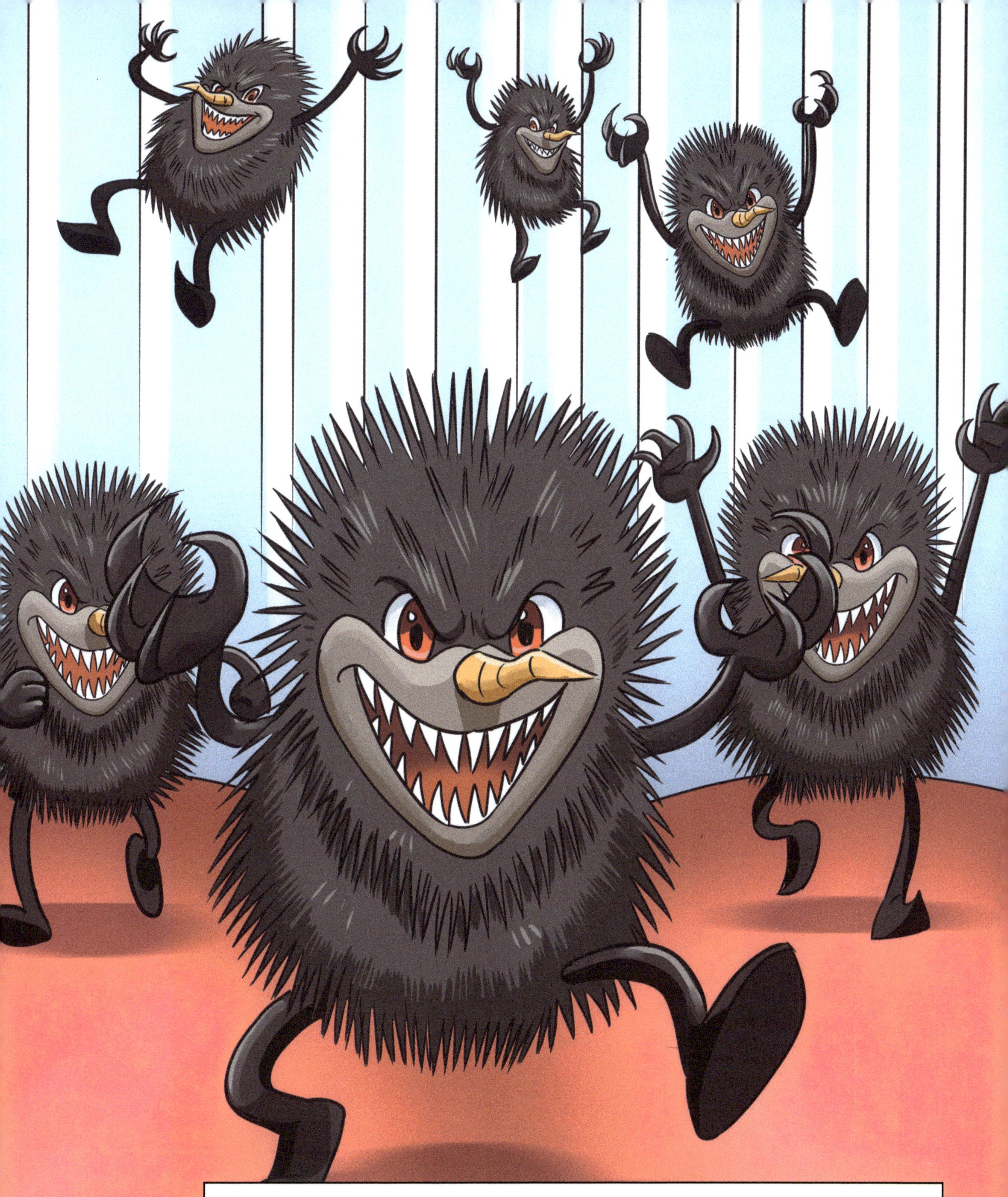

The bacteria in the mouth have fallen under the evil spell of Dental Disease. They have been commanded to destroy all the teeth in Bobby's mouth.

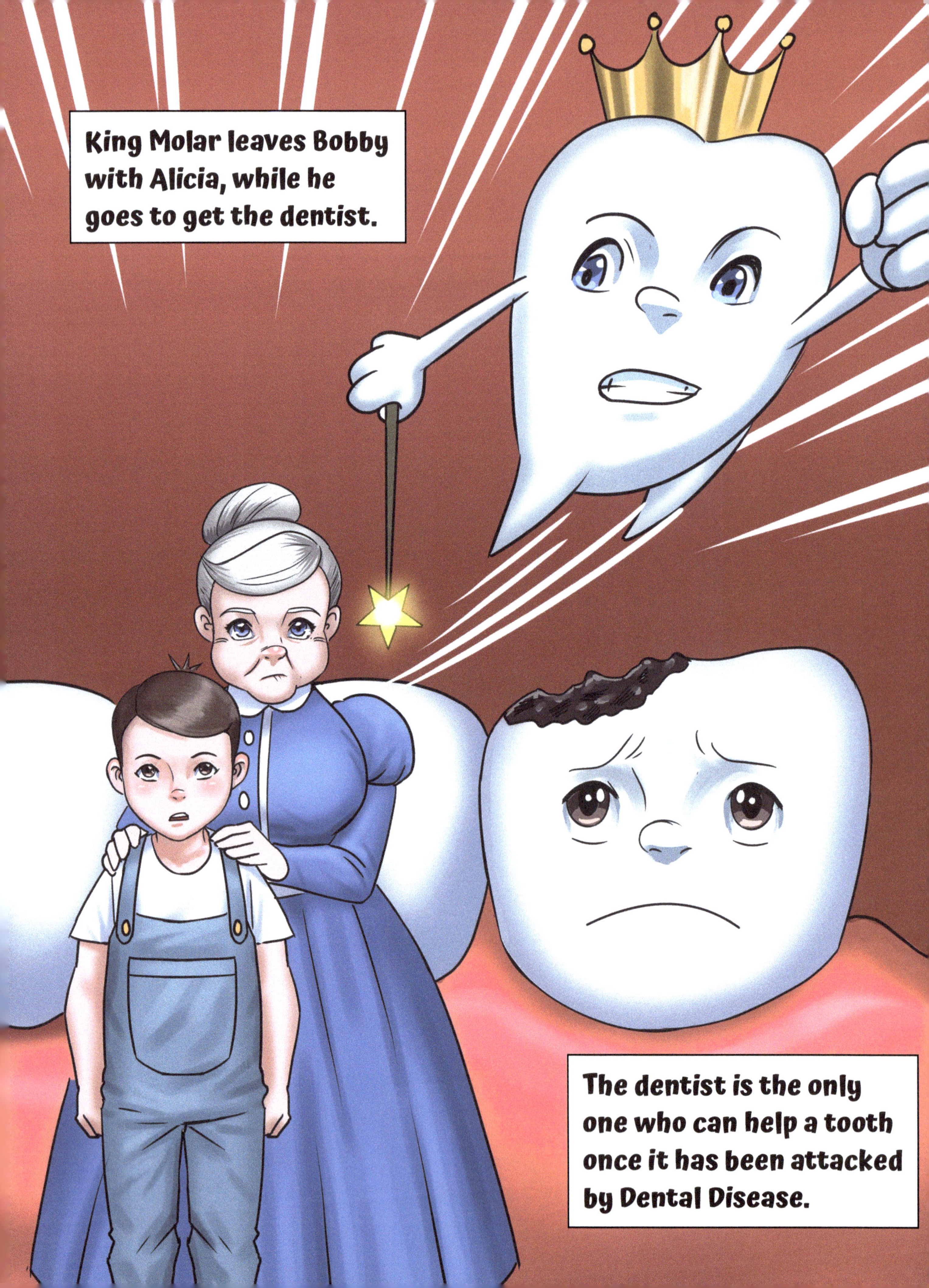

King Molar leaves Bobby with Alicia, while he goes to get the dentist.
The dentist is the only one who can help a tooth once it has been attacked by Dental Disease.

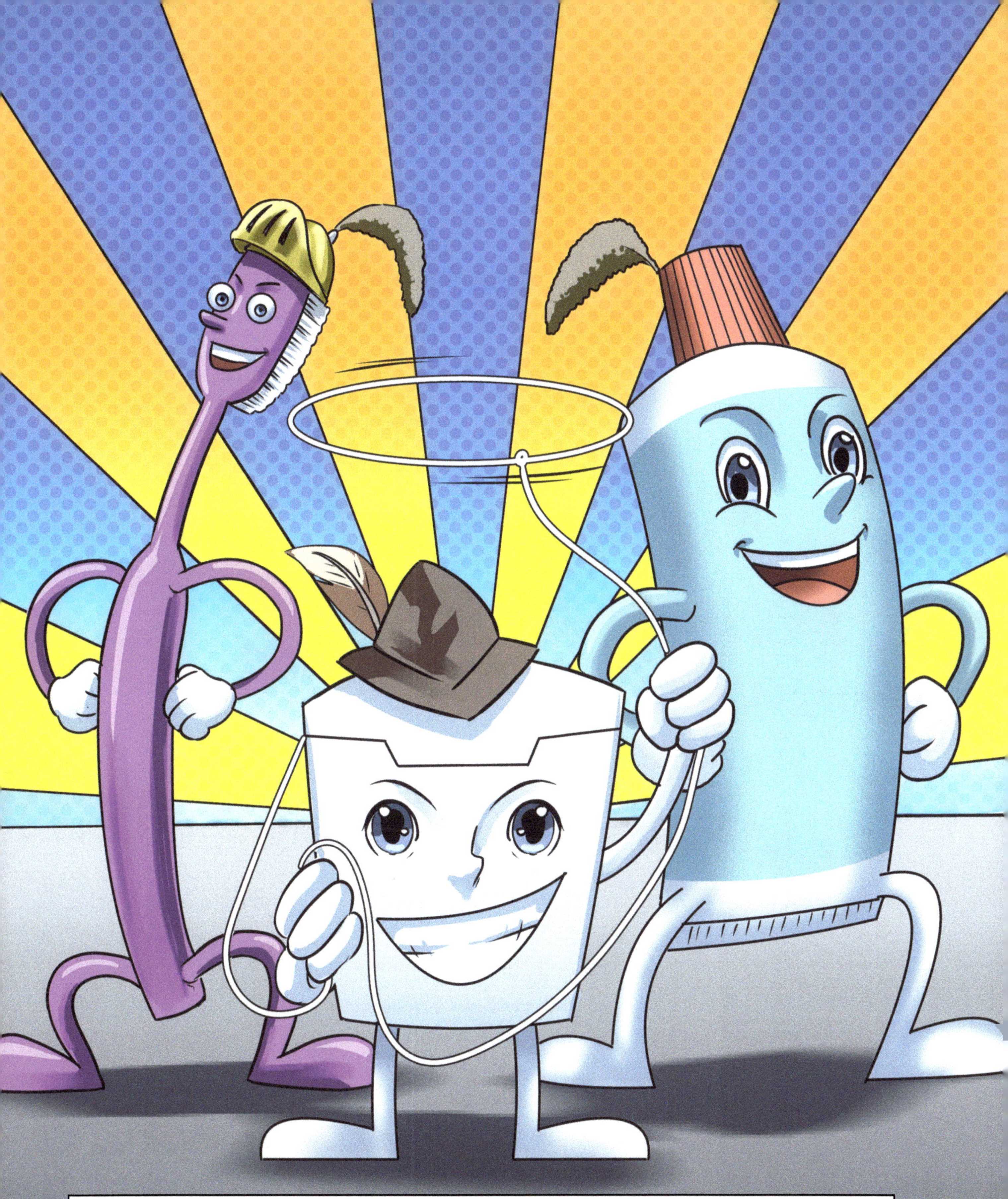

Alicia explains to Bobby that Sir Floss, Sir Brush, and Sir Paste, knights in the King's army, are the best weapons against Dental Disease. "But you must use them regularly."

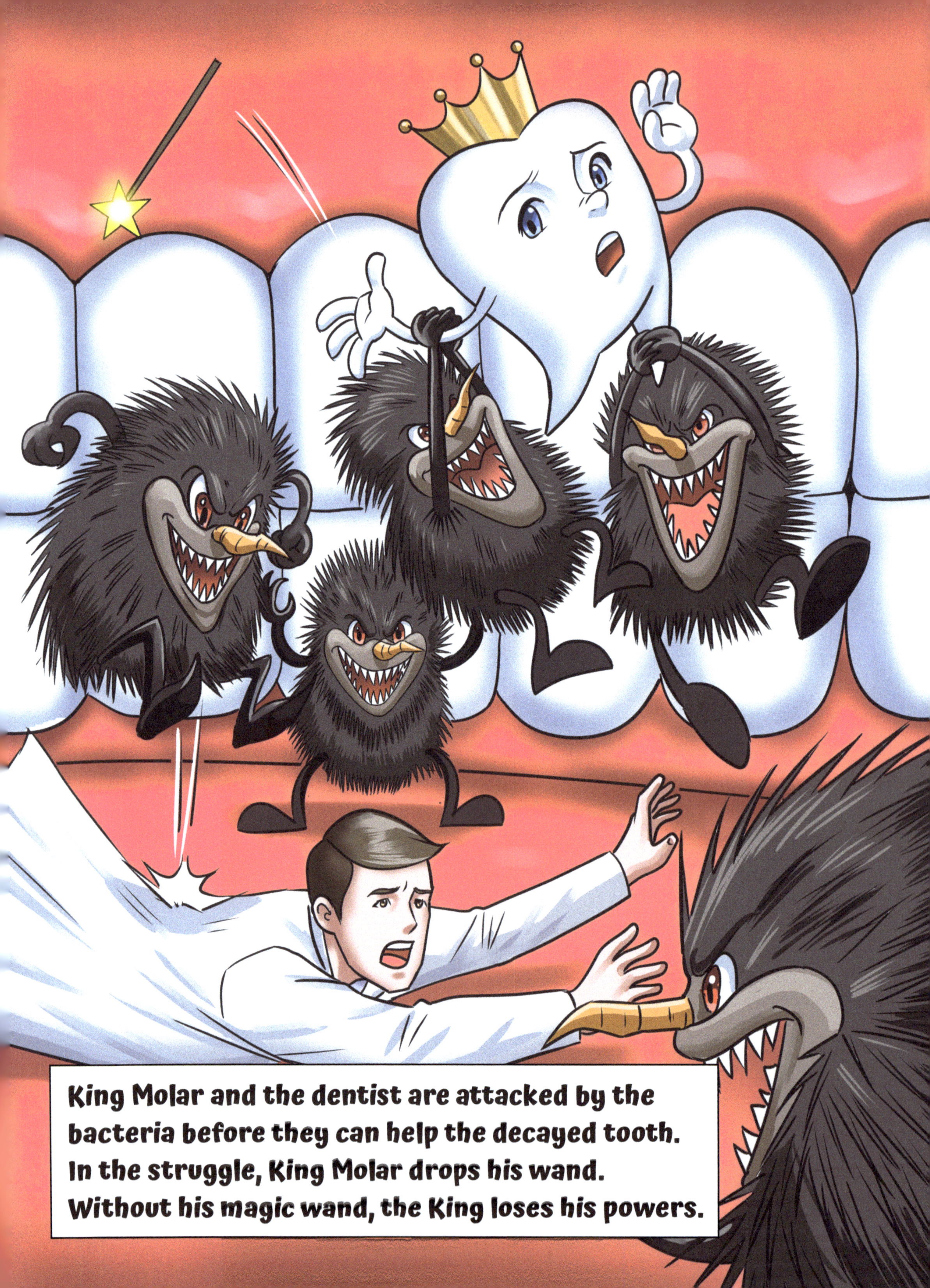

King Molar and the dentist are attacked by the
bacteria before they can help the decayed tooth.
In the struggle, King Molar drops his wand.
Without his magic wand, the King loses his powers.

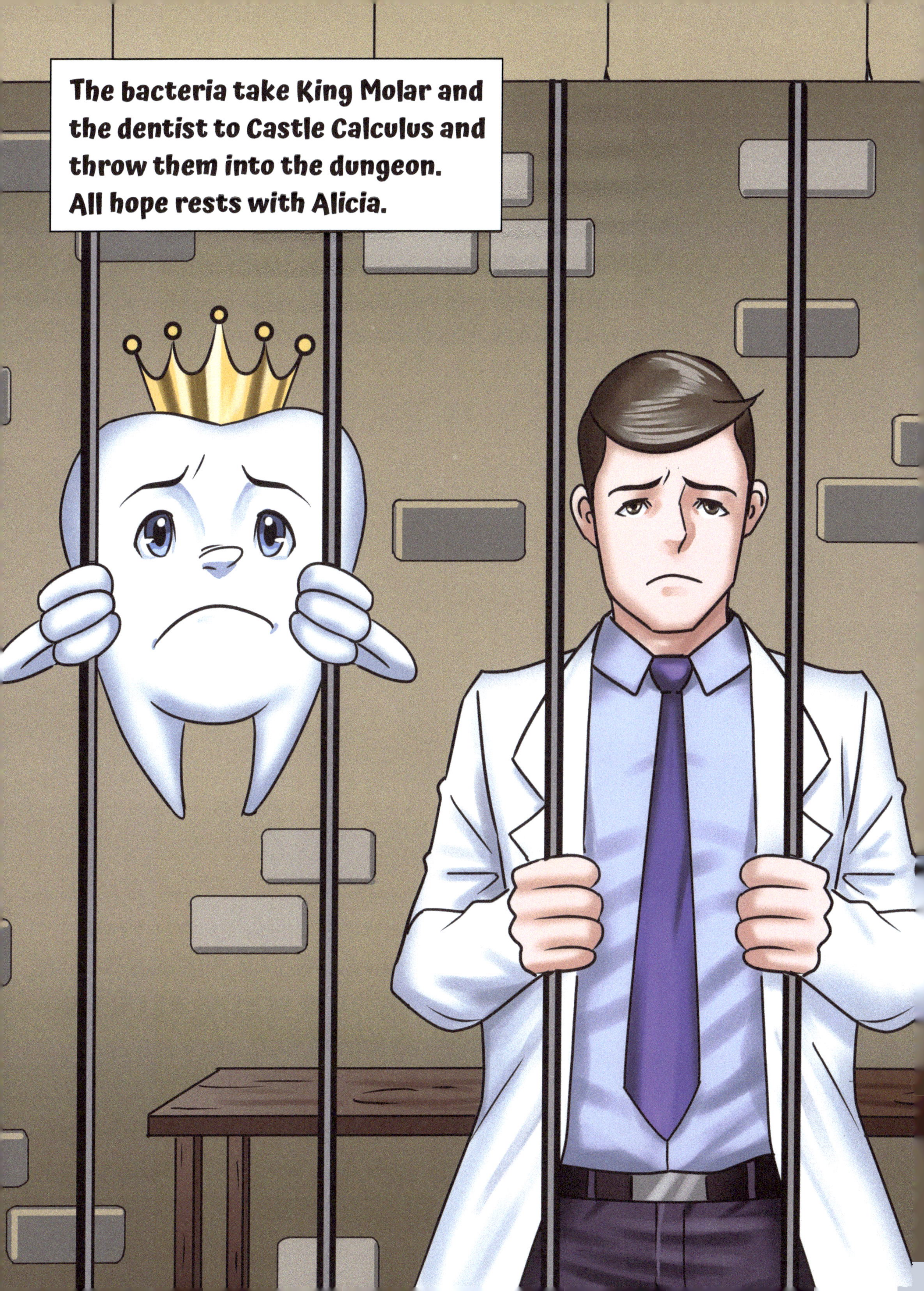
The bacteria take King Molar and the dentist to Castle Calculus and throw them into the dungeon. All hope rests with Alicia.

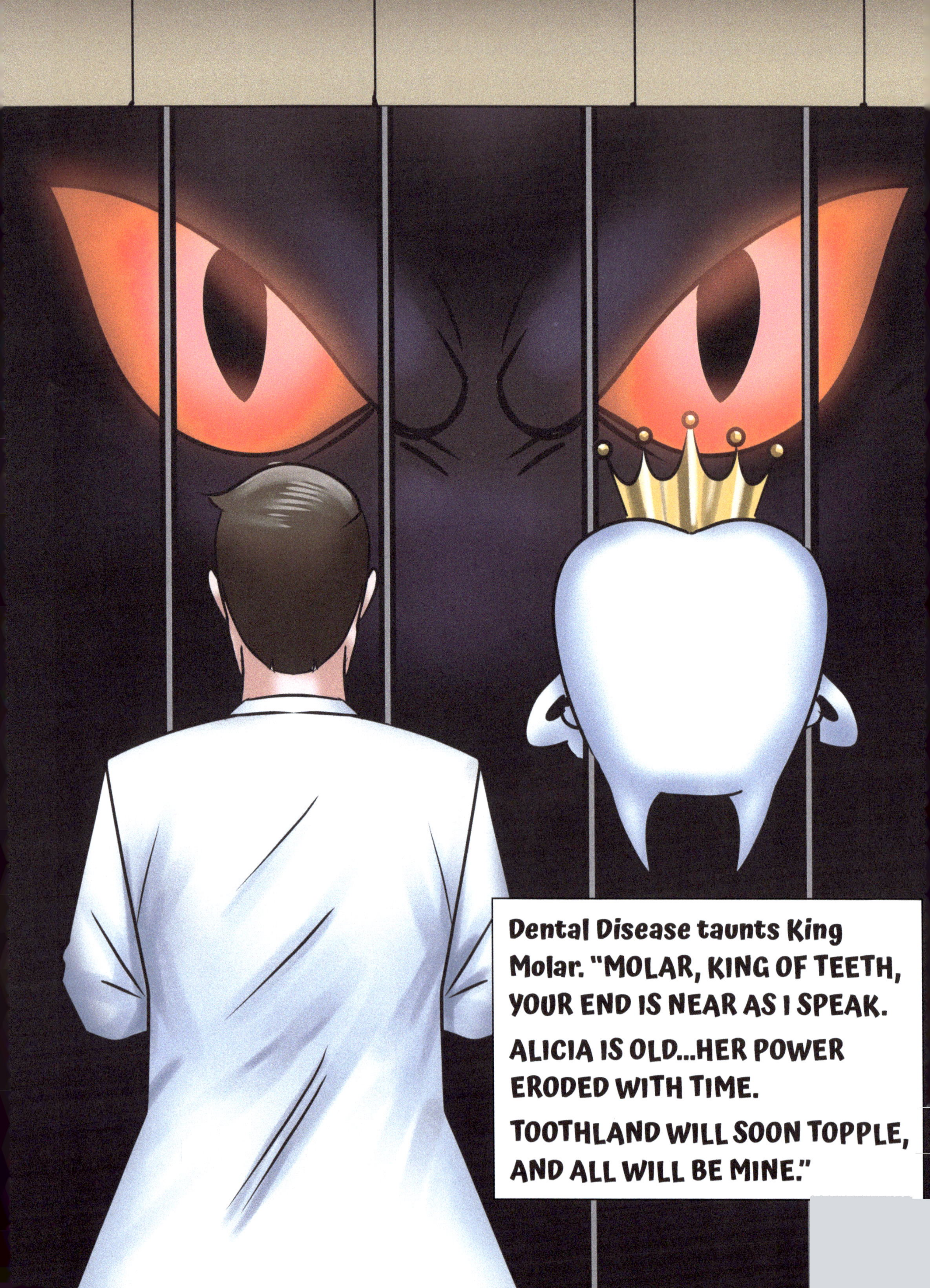

Dental Disease taunts King Molar. "MOLAR, KING OF TEETH, YOUR END IS NEAR AS I SPEAK.

ALICIA IS OLD...HER POWER ERODED WITH TIME.

TOOTHLAND WILL SOON TOPPLE, AND ALL WILL BE MINE."

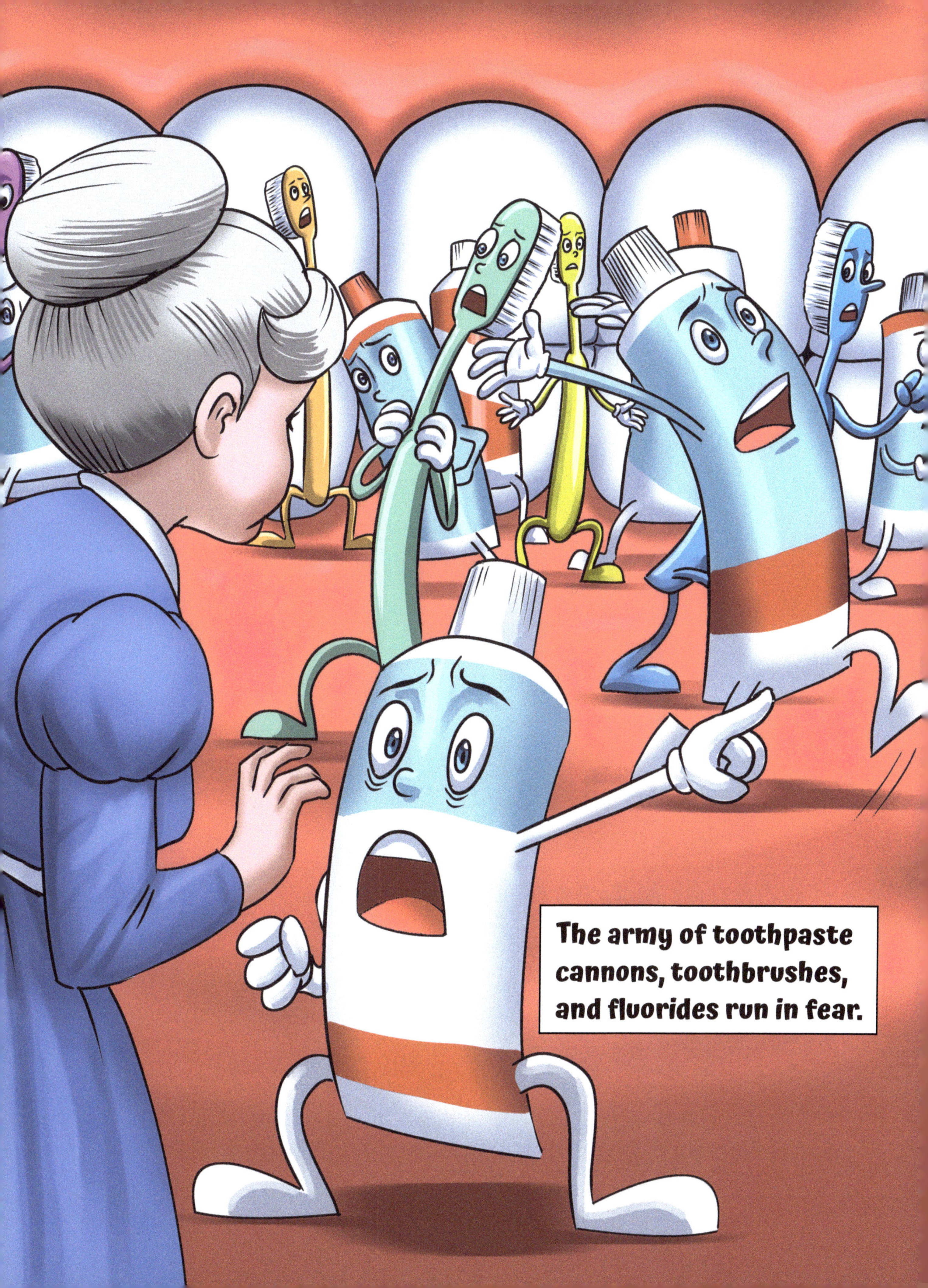
The army of toothpaste cannons, toothbrushes, and fluorides run in fear.

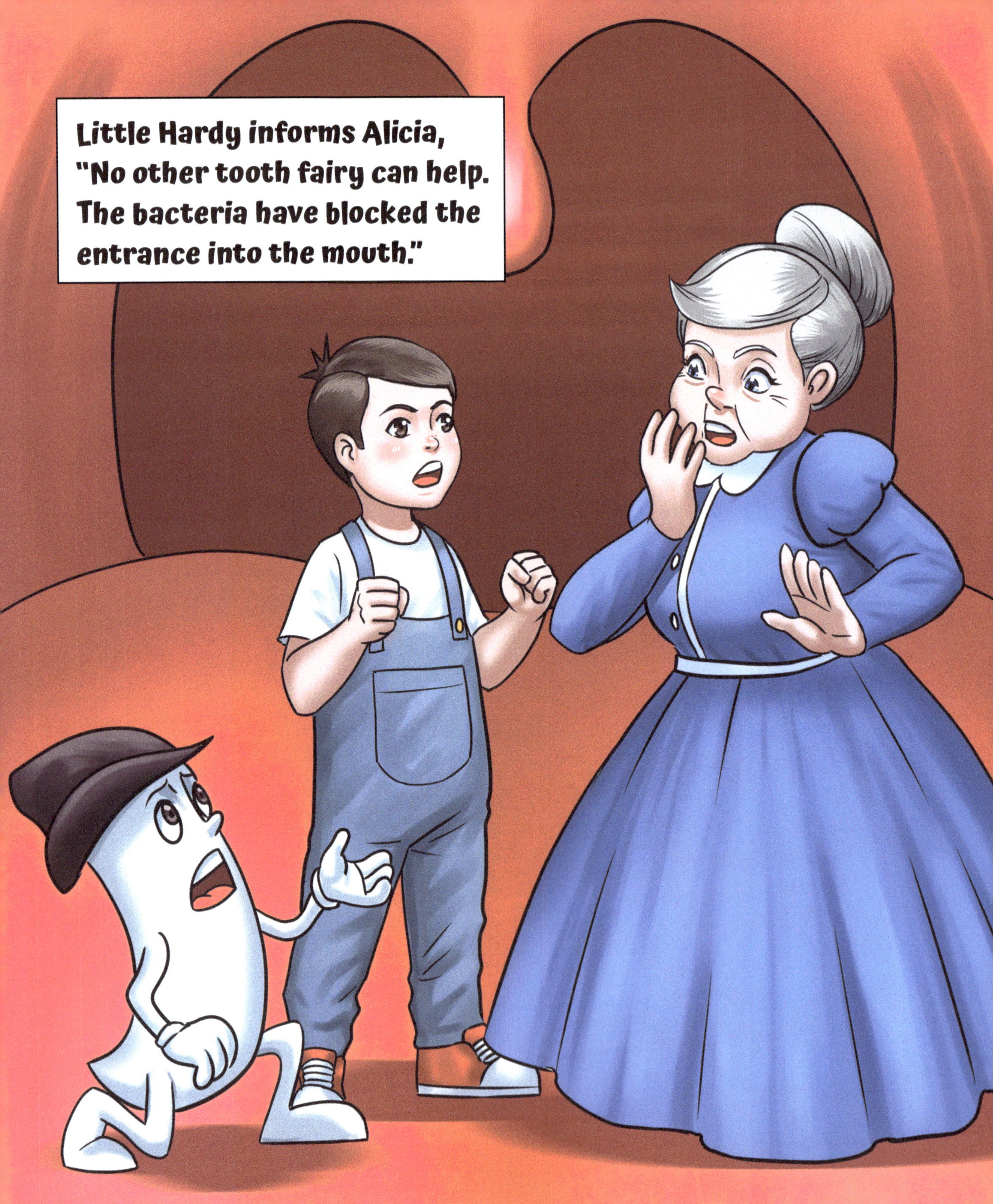

Little Hardy informs Alicia, "No other tooth fairy can help. The bacteria have blocked the entrance into the mouth."
Alicia is frightened. Bobby tells her it could be her big chance. She must lead the fight against Dental Disease.

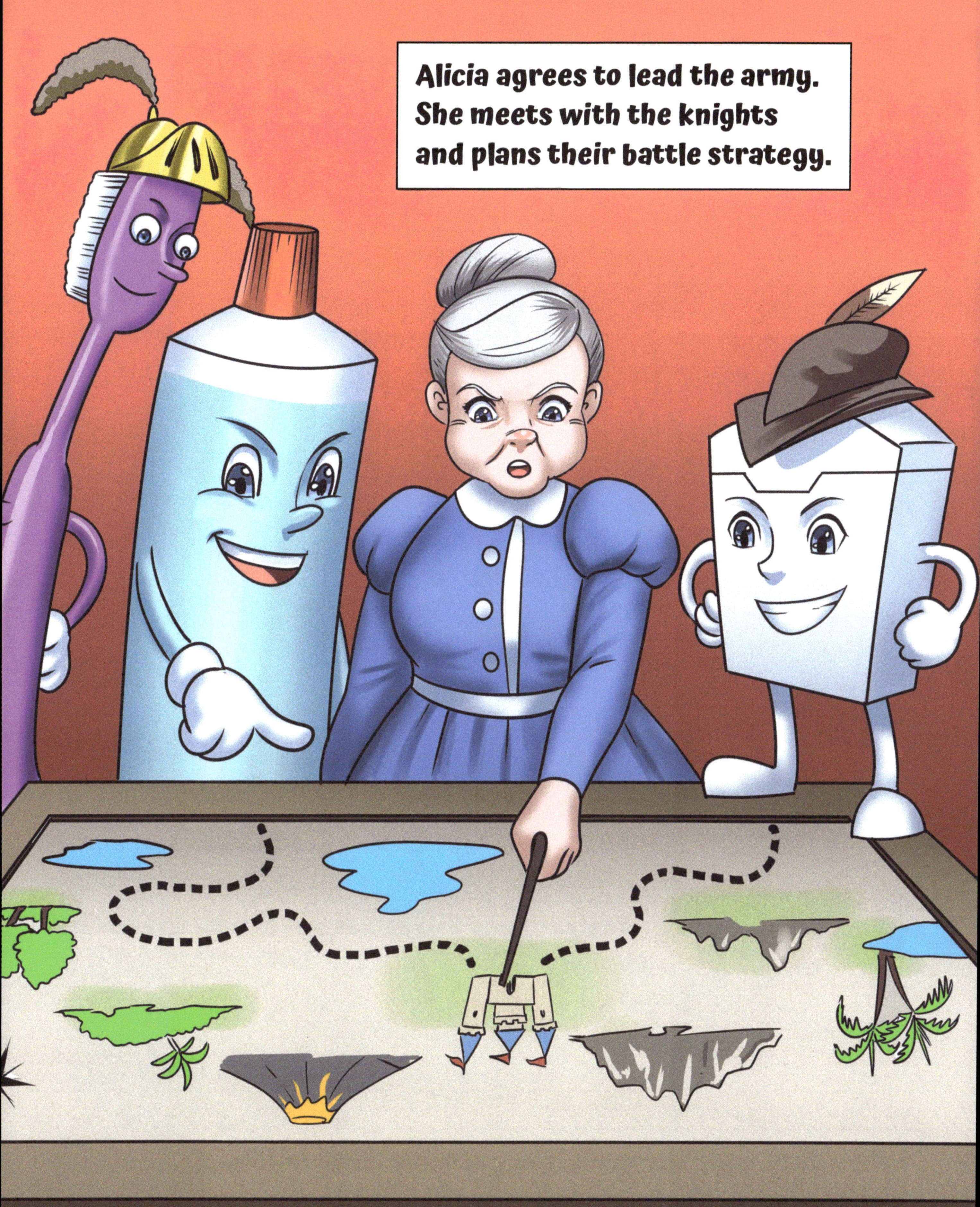

Alicia agrees to lead the army.
She meets with the knights
and plans their battle strategy.

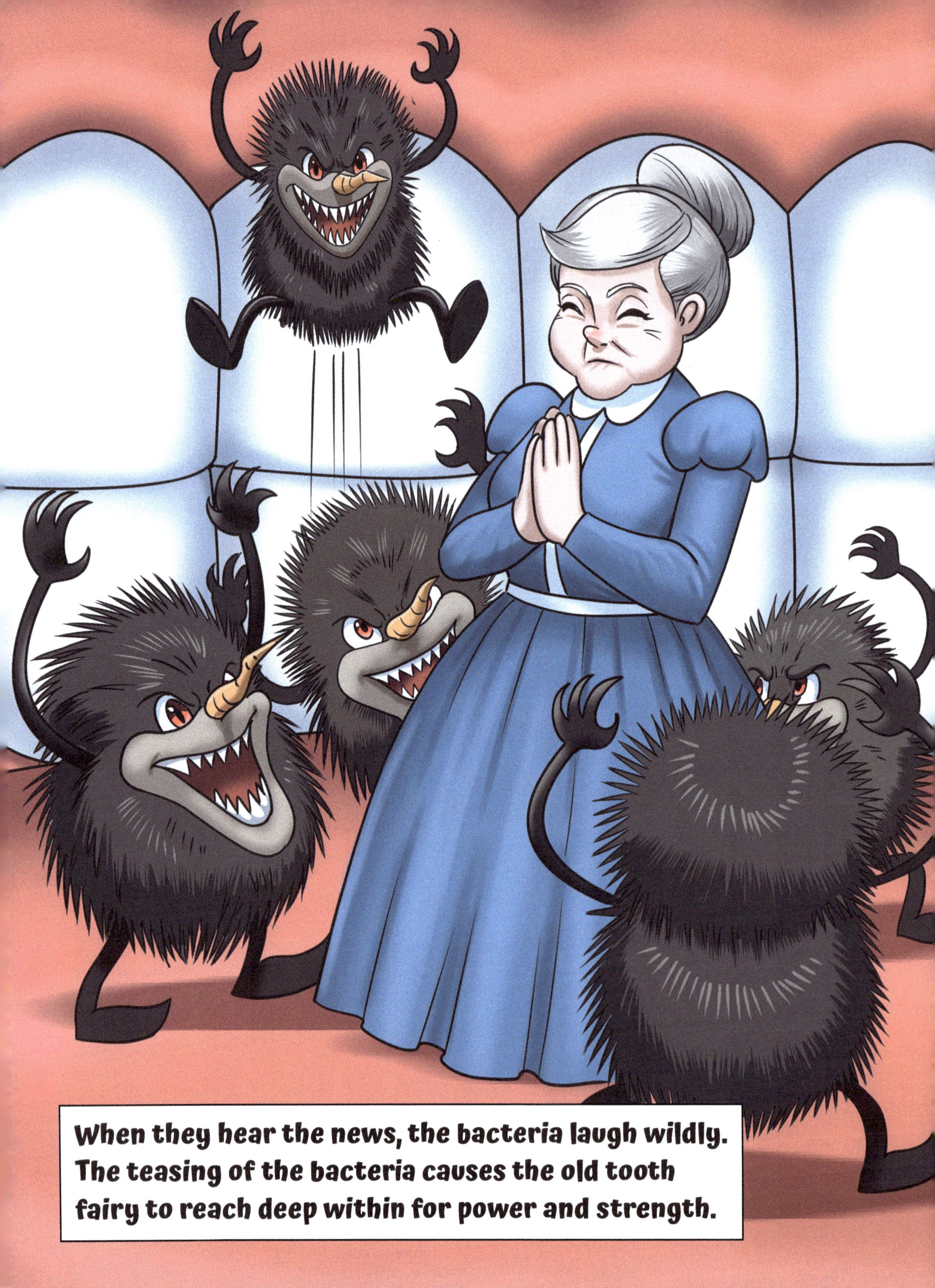

When they hear the news, the bacteria laugh wildly. The teasing of the bacteria causes the old tooth fairy to reach deep within for power and strength.

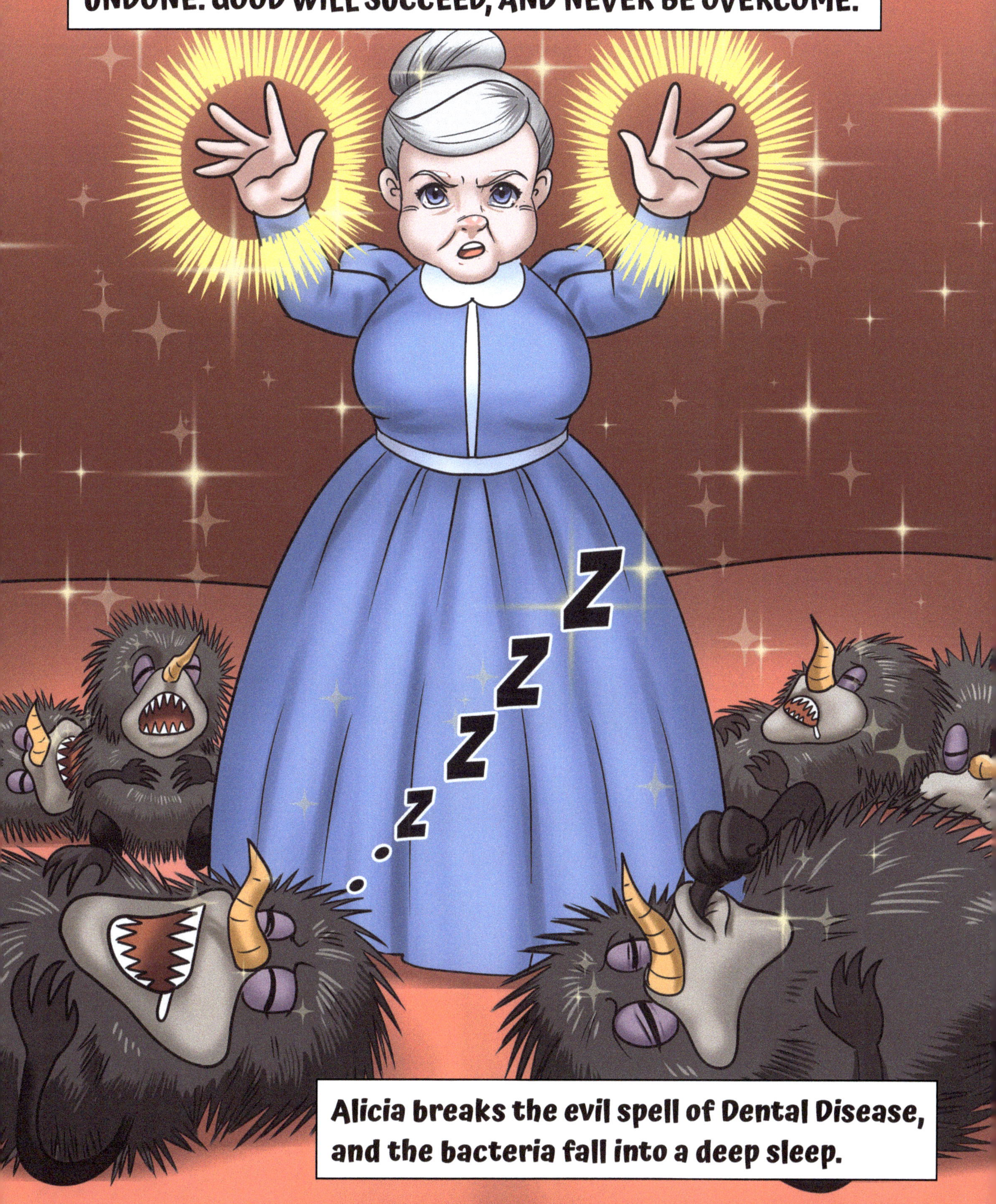

Alicia breaks the evil spell of Dental Disease, and the bacteria fall into a deep sleep.

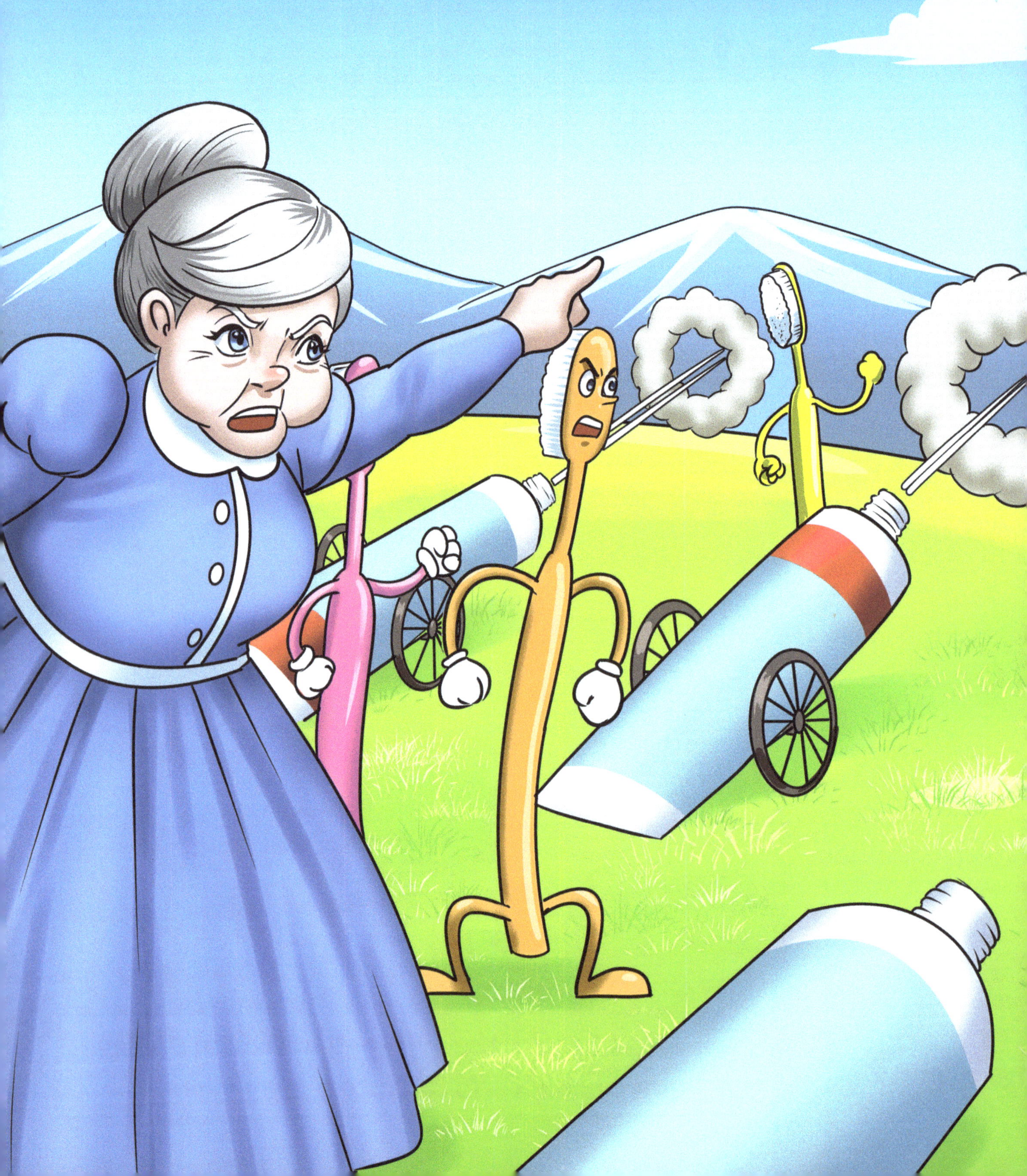

Alicia orders the toothpaste cannons to fire.
The battle has begun. She orders scalers
to break up the main gate of the castle.

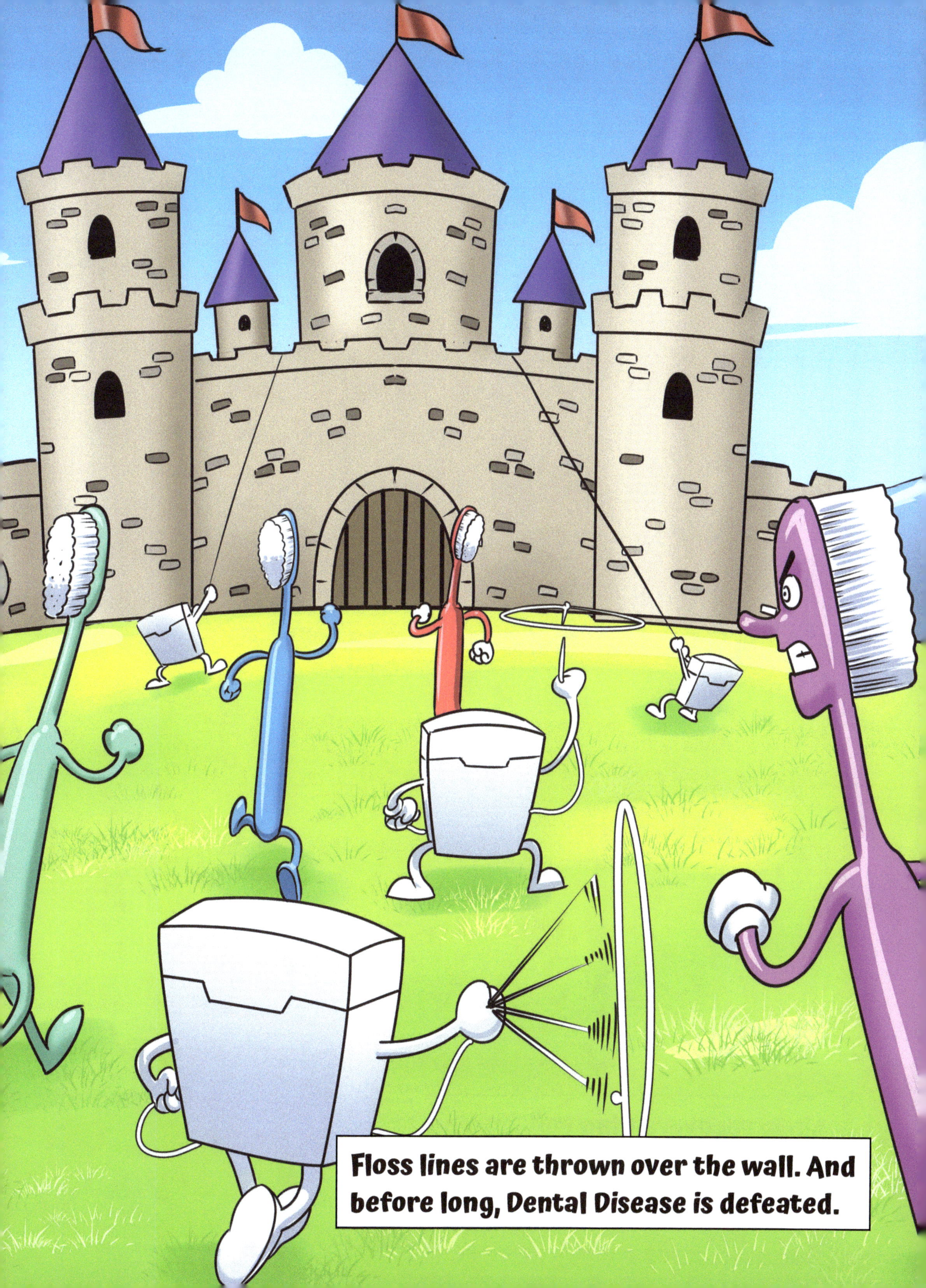
Floss lines are thrown over the wall. And before long, Dental Disease is defeated.

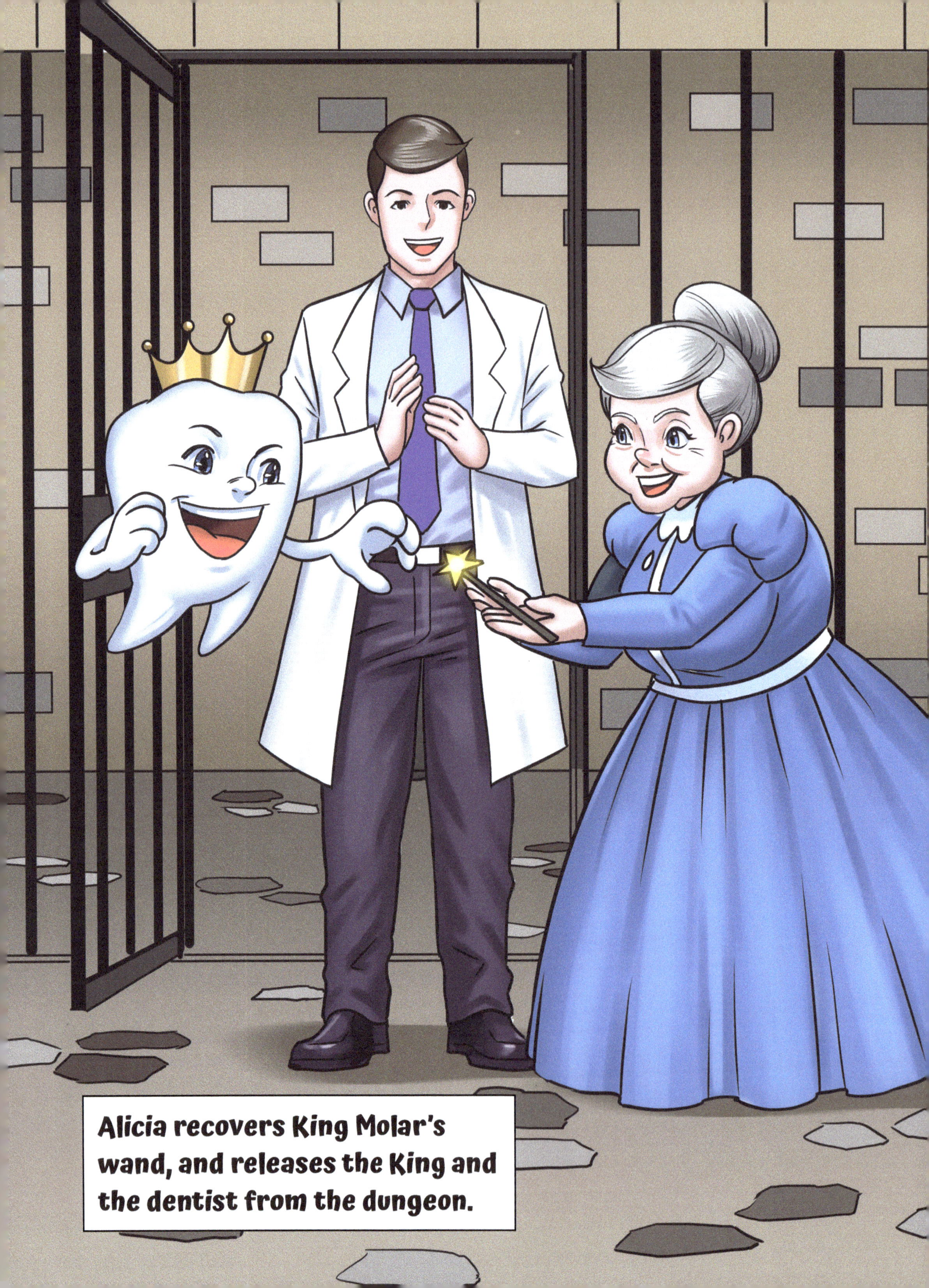

Alicia recovers King Molar's wand, and releases the King and the dentist from the dungeon.

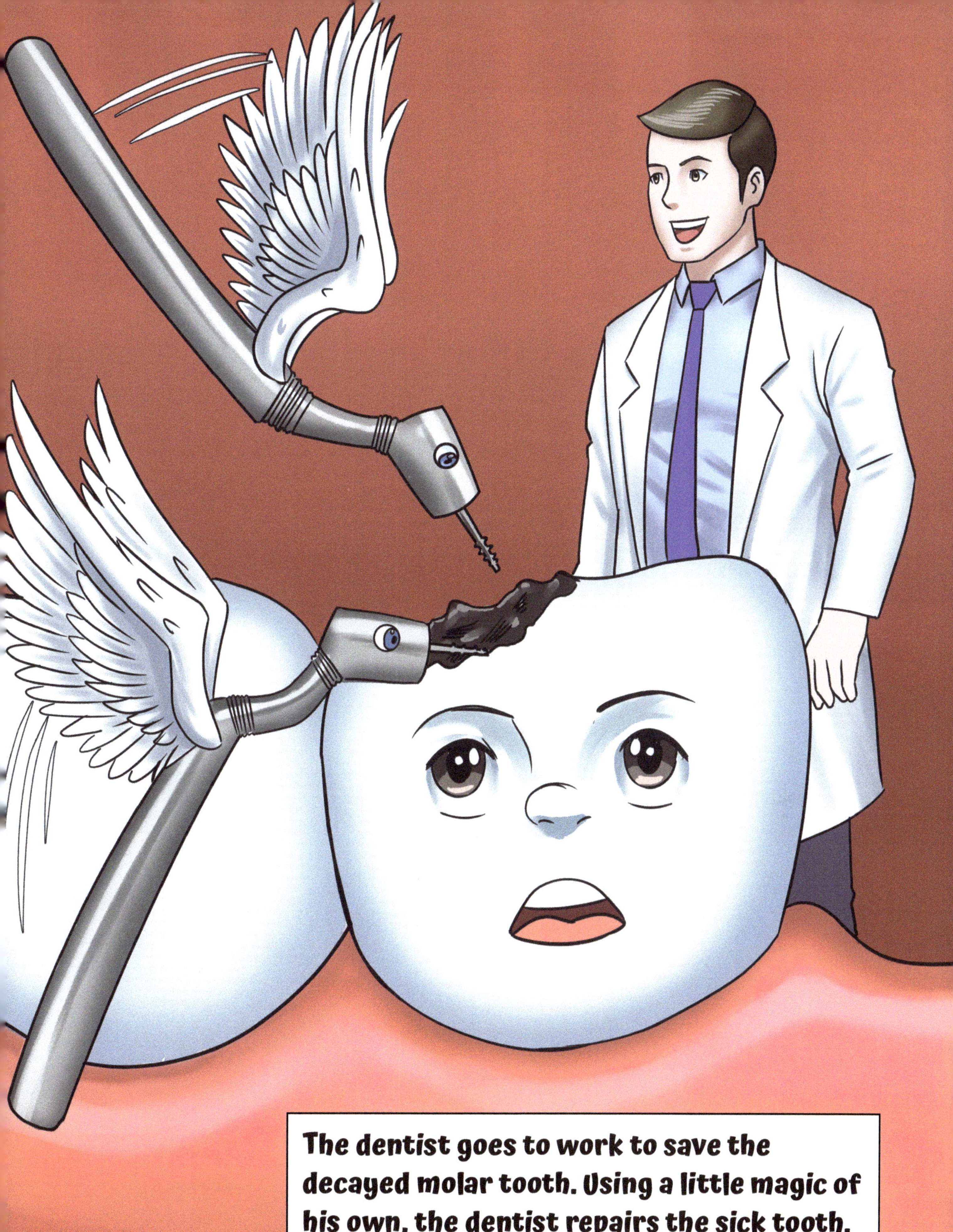

The dentist goes to work to save the decayed molar tooth. Using a little magic of his own, the dentist repairs the sick tooth.

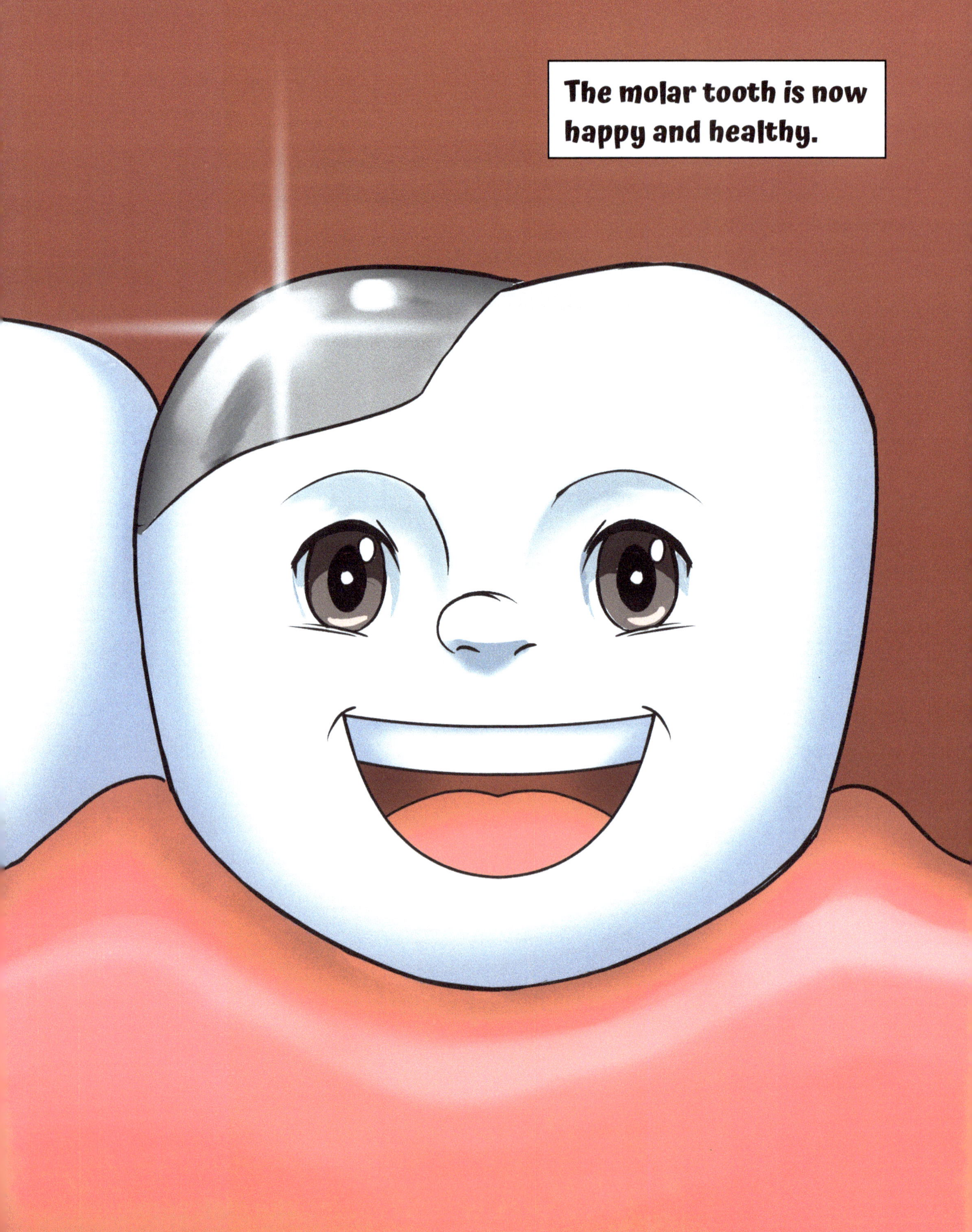
The molar tooth is now happy and healthy.

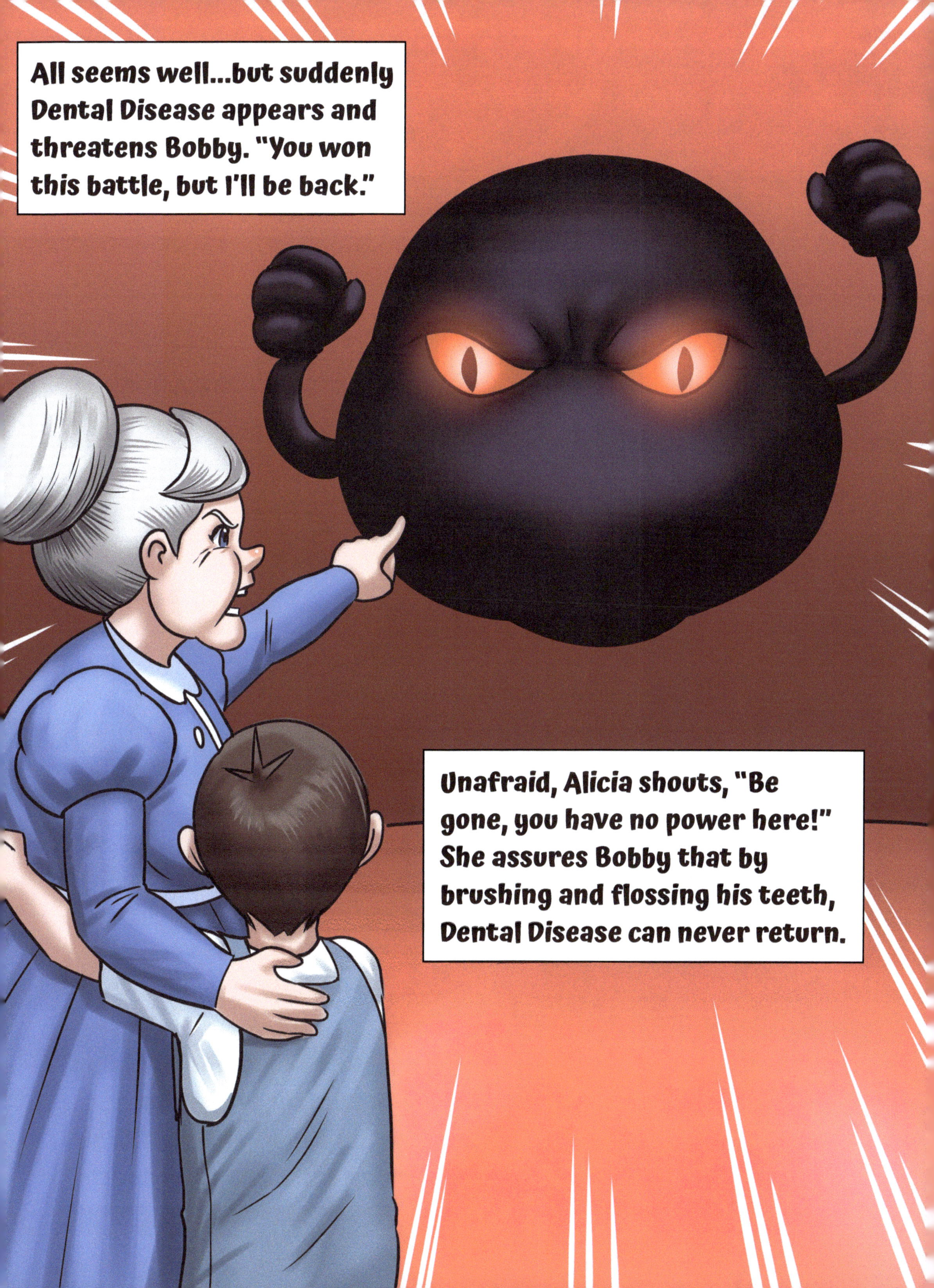

All seems well...but suddenly Dental Disease appears and threatens Bobby. "You won this battle, but I'll be back."
Unafraid, Alicia shouts, "Be gone, you have no power here!" She assures Bobby that by brushing and flossing his teeth, Dental Disease can never return.

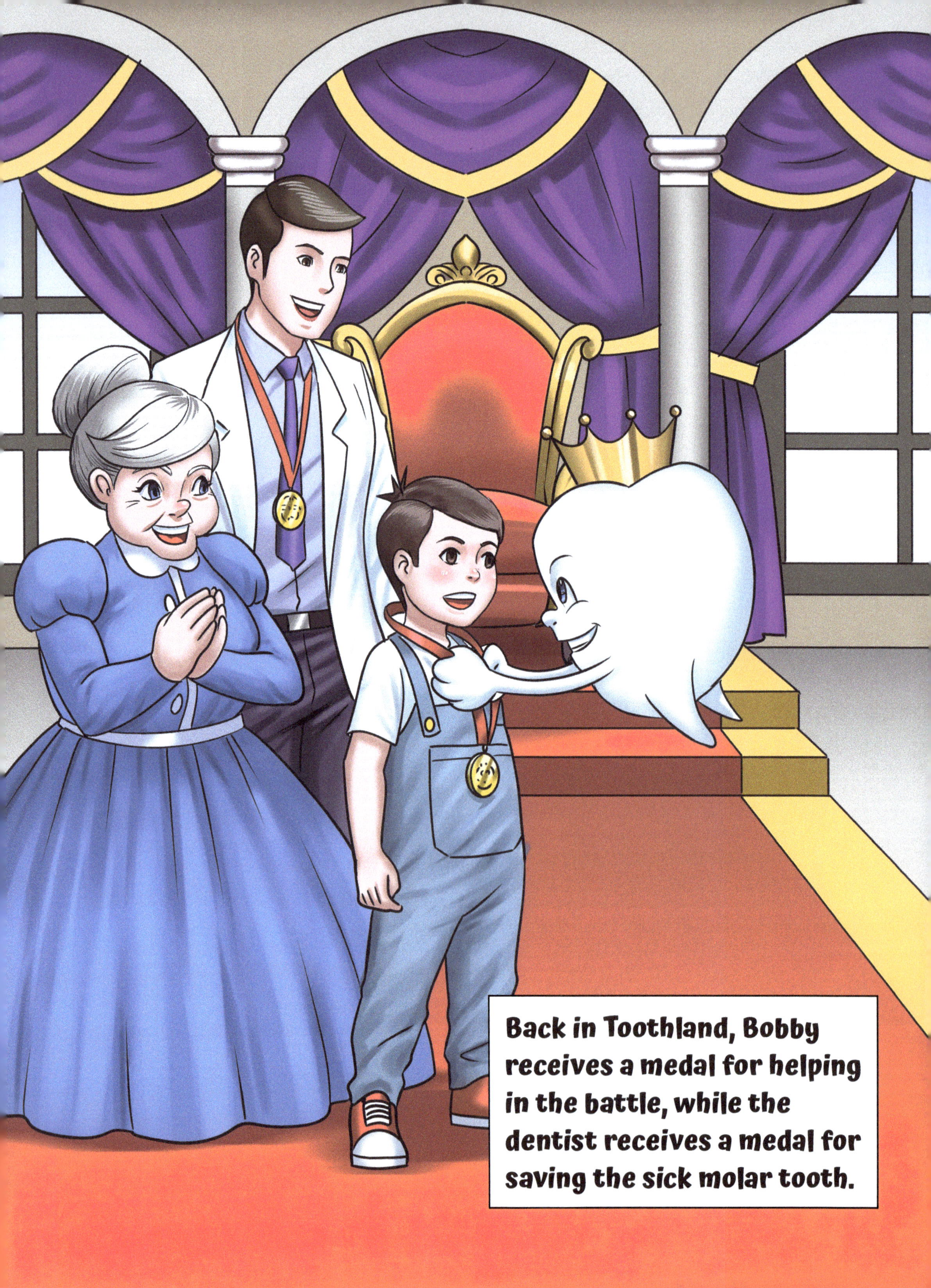

Back in Toothland, Bobby receives a medal for helping in the battle, while the dentist receives a medal for saving the sick molar tooth.

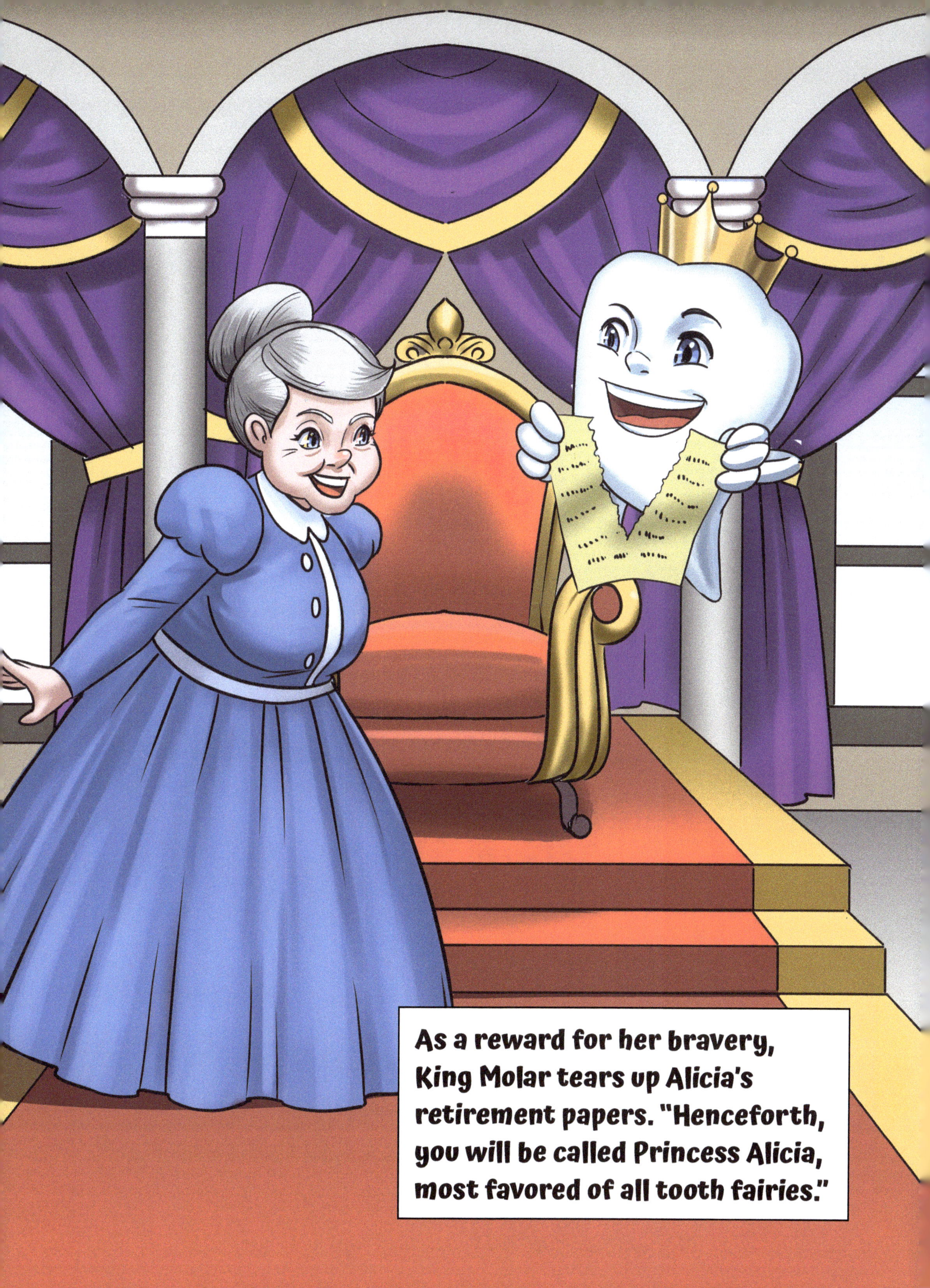
As a reward for her bravery, King Molar tears up Alicia's retirement papers. "Henceforth, you will be called Princess Alicia, most favored of all tooth fairies."

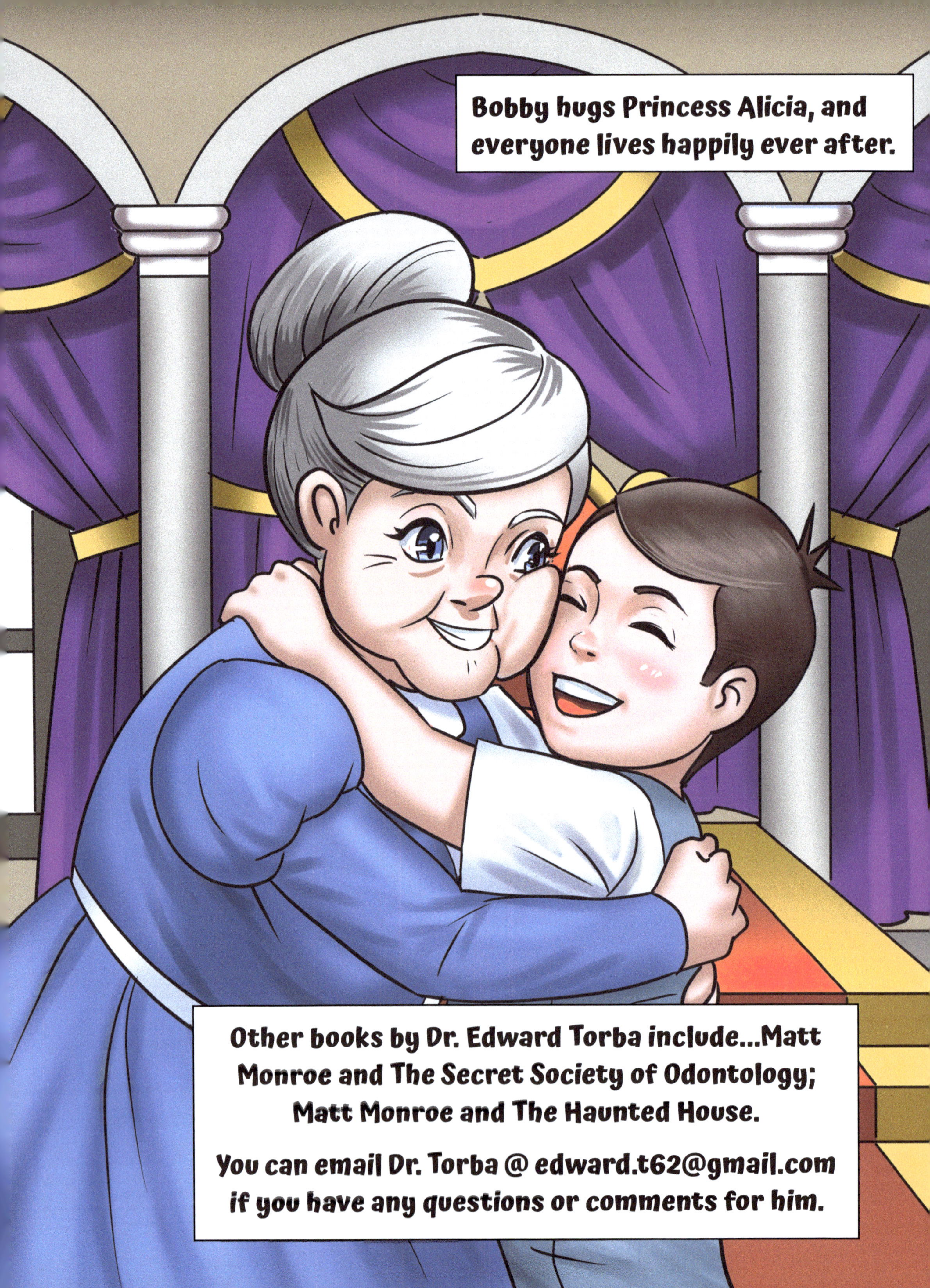

Bobby hugs Princess Alicia, and everyone lives happily ever after.

Other books by Dr. Edward Torba include...Matt Monroe and The Secret Society of Odontology; Matt Monroe and The Haunted House.

You can email Dr. Torba @ edward.t62@gmail.com if you have any questions or comments for him.